Bright Star Woman

Reiki Yoga Manual

Mercedes Déziel-Hupé

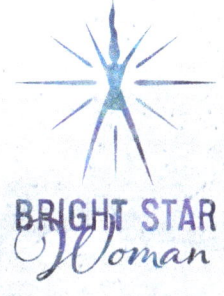

BRIGHT STAR
Woman

Copyright © 2023 by Mercedes Déziel-Hupé

Photographer - Alicia Riddle

All rights reserved.

No part of this book may be reproduced in any form or by any electronic or mechanical means, including information storage and retrieval systems, without written permission from the author, except for the use of brief quotations in a book review.

Please consult your trusted health care provider before starting any mental and/or physical health and wellness practice or program.

The word "healing", as it is used in this book, is meant to refer to the process of cultivating and/or returning to a state of wellness (homeostasis) and a lifestyle of harmony (healthy and life-honouring practices), and is not, in any way, a "cure" claim.

The information in this book is not intended for diagnosis or treatment, but merely as a support to your holistic wellness journey. You are recognizing your role and responsibility in your own well-being, and that the author of this manual can not be held liable for any personal or health-related consequence that may arise from following your practice of the program and practices described in this manual.

Namaste.

Nebula watercolor cover art and watercolor meditation visuals by Mercedes Déziel-Hupé.

ENGLISH: 978-1-7389699-0-6 Bright Star Woman Reiki Yoga Manual
FRENCH: 978-1-7389699-1-3 Manuel de reiki yoga de Bright Star Woman

CONTENTS

DISCLAIMER	vii
ACKNOWLEDGMENTS	ix
AUTHOR'S NOTE	xi
INTRODUCTION	xv

Part I
A POWERFUL HYBRID

WHAT IS REIKI?	3
MEDITATION & RELAXATION	4
REIKI PRINCIPLES & DAILY AFFIRMATION	6
TRADITIONAL REIKI PRINCIPLES	7
BRIGHT STAR WOMAN REIKI PRINCIPLES	8
ATTUNEMENTS	8
WHAT IS YOGA?	13
COMBINING REIKI & YOGA	15
THE BENEFITS OF PRACTISING REIKI YOGA	17
REIKI & THERAPEUTIC TOUCH: THE SOMATIC EFFECT	19
ENERGY AWARENESS & THE SENSES	22
WHO CAN PRACTISE REIKI YOGA?	25
MOST SUITABLE YOGA STYLES	28
HANDS: HEALING PORTALS	30
MUDRAS	30
MERIDIANS AND REFLEXOLOGY	31
PART 1 HIGHLIGHTS	33

Part II
SHAPE YOUR PRACTICE

STRUCTURING YOUR REIKI YOGA PRACTICE	37
GROUNDING & INTENTION	
REIKI ACTIVATION	39
SCANNING YOUR BODY & ENERGY FIELD	41
SELF-TREATMENT	42
HAND POSITIONS	43
MOVEMENT AND ASANAS	52
BREATH AND MEDITATION	55
SOUND: FROM YOGA TO REIKI, CHANTING AND MUSIC	58
INTEGRATION AND GRATITUDE	66
PART 2 HIGHLIGHTS	67
CONSIDERATIONS FOR YOUR REIKI YOGA PRACTICE	68
MINDFULNESS AND VIPASSANA	68
CHAKRAS	69
LIGHT AND COLOURS	70
HYDRATION AND THE WATER CONNECTION	74

Part III
SEQUENCES TO BUILD UPON

REIKI YOGA SEQUENCES	79
SEQUENCE 1: GROUNDING	80
PRACTICE FOCUS BY AREA: LEGS & HIPS	
SEQUENCE 2: FEELING	101
PRACTICE FOCUS BY AREA: BACK & TORSO	
SEQUENCE 3: OPENING/LIGHTENING/ EXPANDING	120
PRACTICE FOCUS BY AREA: HEAD, NECK, & SHOULDERS	
PART 3 HIGHLIGHTS	142

Part IV
THE JOURNEY

ENERGY HEALING MEDITATIONS	145
MOTHER EARTH PINK HEART MEDITATION	145
BRIGHT STAR WOMAN – STAR HEART MEDITATION	146
KUNDALINI YOGA MEDITATIONS FOR HEALING	148
COMPLEMENTARY PRACTICES	152
Working with Energy	
HEALING THE FEMININE	153
DEVELOPING INTUITION	156
CARING FOR OUR BODY	157
AN ENVIRONMENT THAT SUPPORTS YOUR PRACTICE	160
THE ETHICS OF SHARING & TEACHING REIKI YOGA	164
PART 4 HIGHLIGHTS	168
LIVING YOUR REIKI YOGA	169
PRAISE FOR BRIGHT STAR WOMAN REIKI YOGA MANUAL	171
ABOUT THE AUTHOR	173
REFERENCES FOR FURTHER EXPLORATION	175
BOOKS BY TOPIC	177

DISCLAIMER

Please consult your trusted health care provider before starting any mental and/or physical health and wellness practice or program.

The word "healing", as it is used in this book, is meant to refer to the process of cultivating and/or returning to a state of wellness (homeostasis) and a lifestyle of harmony (healthy and life-honouring practices), and is not, in any way, a "cure" claim.

The information in this book is not intended for diagnosis or treatment, but merely as a support to your holistic wellness journey. You are recognizing your role and responsibility in your own well-being, and that the author of this manual can not be held liable for any personal or health-related consequence that may arise from following your practice of the program and practices described in this manual.

Namaste.

ACKNOWLEDGMENTS

Expressing gratitude is an empowering practice, much like Reiki yoga. This book wouldn't have come to life without the help, support, and expertise of many kind and gifted people.

Thank you to my son, Gaspard, for being a bright light of pure love and healing. By your presence, you remind me of what matters and who I am. Thank you to my son, Hervé, who was in my womb while I wrote this book, for reminding me of the miracle of life and the wonderful healing power of Reiki yoga and meditation. Thank you to my daughter, Clémentine, for gifting me further healing and empowerment with your birth. Thank you three beautiful souls for each day that grace me with your love and light. I love you three to the moon and back, and I feel blessed that you chose me as your mama.

Thank you to my husband, Scott, for supporting me emotionally and practically by holding down the family fort, any time I dedicated to writing. Thank you for being a great dad and partner. You made this dream possible, thank you. I love you.

Thank you to my mom, Carolyn, who introduced me to Reiki when I was 18 years old. That workshop has changed my relationship to energy and healing, and ultimately, it's changed my life.

Thank you to my two early readers, friends, and mentors, Marie-Claude and Tatiana, for providing constructive feedback and unbridled encouragement.

Thank you to my family and friends, who cheered me on and told me to "just write." Thank you to my Reiki clients and yoga students, who believed I was sharing something of value, worth spreading widely.

Thank you to my early Reiki and yoga teachers for sharing these beautiful healing practices and inspiring me to pursue these respective paths.

Thank you to Alicia, my gifted photographer, who helped me bring the sequences to life through images.

And last but not least, thank you to my designer, Kayla Curry, for understanding my vision and rendering it beautifully.

AUTHOR'S NOTE

This manual is born from a passion for wellness, and from years of dedicated yoga and Reiki practices, independently. I came to realize the value of each modality and their potential combined power. I began to explore ways in which to marry the two practices that had given me so much. Yoga saved me from depression and burnout. Yoga and meditation gave me peace when in the throes of deep grief from my two miscarriages. Reiki empowered me through anxiety and my mother's cancer. Reiki and yoga each have helped me transition as an entrepreneur, healer, and teacher, as well as helped me recover from hypothyroidism, a traumatic birth, and more recently, a pre-diabetic condition.

I introduced Reiki yoga to my students in the winter of 2017 to great reception. The following manual is the result of these experiences, the classes I led, the student feedback I've received, and intuitive guidance to share this ancient wisdom in our contemporary context.

I believe that Reiki is a birthright; we are born with life energy and we innately know when something is out of alignment. Often, we intuitively know how to best treat ourselves, whether this healing is physical, emotional, mental, or spiritual. Children know this and practise Reiki all the time! In fact, children will instinctively place their hands on a "bobo" (theirs or someone else's) to make it feel better, touch their own sore belly, or "pet" a parent or friend if they feel their energy is sad, out of sorts, or "low" vibrationally. As adults, we just need to be reminded how to listen to our own guidance, how to trust ourselves and Spirit/Creator/God/Universe for giving us such empowering tools.

What I share in this book is based largely on personal and professional experience, studies, and books I have read on Reiki, yoga, and meditation, and on testimonials from my clients and students. I've included resources to help further your exploration and learning but have deliberately chosen to forego a traditional bibliography.

Practising Reiki yoga does not require any training, it only requires openness; you need space and time to allow yourself to be, to receive messages from your body and your higher self, the wisest part of you. It is similar to yogic philosophy; you do not need training to practise yoga, but you do need training and experience to teach it. The same applies to the practice of Reiki, and of Reiki yoga.

I would recommend yoga teachers who would like to integrate Reiki yoga into their classes to pursue formal Reiki training. Just as the yoga industry needs trained professionals, so does the Reiki world; it is a question of respect for the disciplines, and a matter of safety and integrity for both students and teachers. Training in Reiki will enable a teacher to understand the modality they are sharing and will allow them to offer Reiki hands-on to their yoga students, adding value to their current yogic hands-on adjustments (or assists).

I hope you will welcome this practice and continue to explore it as you embark on your journey of self-discovery, wellness and holistic healing.

Reiki blessings, Shanti Om.

Mercedes Déziel-Hupé
Bright Star Woman

INTRODUCTION

I was initiated into Usui Reiki at 18, when my mother invited me to a Reiki attunement workshop, offered by Deborah Fish, M.Sc.. Deborah was a practising psychotherapist who had added alternative healing methods to her practice, from Reiki to hypnotherapy and tapping (Emotional Freedom Technique – EFT). That fateful afternoon, my eyes and heart were open along with my Reiki channel.

In a group of women, I received Reiki life force energy for the first time. I also felt something shift and open within me. As I was being attuned, the top of my head seemed to expand, my feet rooted down, my hands warmed and buzzed, and my whole body energized. I felt the difference between channelling and receiving Reiki energy; in the former, I allowed the energy to flow through me, and in the latter, I allowed myself to accept the energy for my own healing. Channelling felt like a gentle buzzing current. Receiving felt like a warm bath enveloping me. Thus, I practised channelling and receiving the white light of Reiki with my fellow initiate practitioners. Everything felt so awe-inspiring. And though I would not fully commit to my Reiki practice for years, it was the beginning of a life-altering journey of wellness and empowerment.

After years of struggling with my own physical and mental health, with loss, scarcity mindset, and chronic dissatisfaction, namely with my career, I found yoga when I was in the heart of my burnout. After dabbling in yoga's physical practice since I was a teenager, I came to realize the transformative power of mindfulness through a regular yoga practice and integrating yogic philosophy principles. I'd been working unusually long hours on a cycle that seemed relentless, and I felt unsatisfied and misunderstood. Ultimately, it was the wrong fit for me professionally and personally. I could try to blame my circumstances on external factors, or I could take stock of my life and the choices that brought me to that point. It was a bumpy road to recovery, in body and soul, but I was aware.

I wanted to heal, and I wanted to be happy. Through trial and error, attempting to change the shape of my life through ill-fitting career choices, I finally decided to pursue my hatha yoga 200-hour teacher training. Initially, I wasn't sure I even wanted to teach in the traditional studio setting, but discovered I loved to share the fruits of my learning. I graduated just weeks after turning 30 and then began a new phase of my life, health, and career. My focus turned to creating and living harmoniously, where wellness and happiness existed as the basis for an intentional, healthful, and abundant life.

Little did I know then that my resolve would be tested with the grief of my first and second miscarriages within the same year... But my vision was to create a life of meaning and harmony, not one of perfection, where there would never be sadness, disappointment, or mistakes. I knew deep down that I wanted to be real, and I wanted to walk my talk. In fact, I'd affirmed to the Universe that I desired this level of alignment, as my final yoga course project was to create a mandala, which I chose to represent "harmony."

With this guiding theme, I started teaching yoga in studios, community centres, and offices, and learning how to apply it to my own everyday. Not surprisingly, I found an affinity for energy-infused yoga styles and an overall therapeutic approach to the practice. I had heard echoes of yoga teachers, who happened to be Reiki practitioners, combining the two practices.

After some research, I noticed that there was very little written on this hybrid style, and there didn't seem to be any guiding principles. It was the Wild West! Keeping in mind the principle of Reiki as a birthright, I decided then to humbly share what I knew with my students to empower them in their wellness journeys. Through inspiration, open student-teacher communication, and hands-on experience, I drew a few guidelines for practising Reiki yoga. Out of a desire to share age-old wisdom in a newer way, in a form that is convenient for contemporary life, yet still connects us with intangible mystery and infinite healing power, this book was born.

The Bright Star Woman Reiki Yoga Manual is named after my spirit name, given to me by a Cree Elder, White Wolf, when I was 27, just a year after the burnout that changed the course of my life. He told me that I was to lead by example, that like the stars, light was my nature and shining was my purpose. Seeing me enlivened and frankly, very proud, he reminded me that there were endless stars in the sky and that each had a purpose. Little did I know at the time what was to come.

In the years that followed, I stepped into my role as a healer, for myself and professionally. I recommitted to my Reiki practice, and started teaching yoga and meditation, all while anchoring my own regular practice. It is these practices that carried me through depression, hypothyroidism, anxiety, grief and loss. They brought me back to my Self, my centre, my peace. Whenever I felt lost or foggy, the wisdom of Reiki, yoga, and meditation gave me clarity and direction. Witnessing the tremendous benefits in my own life, I simply had to share the wonders of these applied teachings.

I believe we are beings of light, living in bodies, and it is our adventure to remember our nature, and our pleasure to shine for ourselves, as well as to give permission to our brothers and sisters to shine their own unique light in the world.

Mercedes may have written this book, but Bright Star Woman inspired it through whispers Mercedes received in meditation, and in her yoga and Reiki practices. Bright Star Woman offered guidance when sharing these teachings with students and clients. Bright Star Woman invites you to rediscover your light and to empower yourself through awareness and practice.

My hope is that this book, or rather its content, will act as a homing beacon for those embodied souls who wish to reclaim their power, regain agency over their lives, health and bodies, and who desire to create a harmonious life of wellness, intention, and meaning, from the inside out. The light of Reiki yoga will bring you home to yourself, by reminding you who you are. And all the better if we can add a little light to our world in the process... Let's shine brighter together!

Part One

A Powerful Hybrid

WHAT IS REIKI?

REIKI IS an ancient Japanese healing art, often credited to Dr Mikao Usui for its (re)discovery at the end of his 21-day meditation on Mount Kurama-yama. The word "Reiki" can be translated to "universal life force energy." It is believed by many Reiki practitioners and historians that the essence of Reiki as a self-healing method was known to Tibetan monks who practised and guarded this modality for hundreds (if not thousands) of years.

Reiki is a holistic practice to help bring your mind, body, and soul to a place of peace, harmony, and alignment. In simplest terms, Reiki is a form of energy work. Often, a practitioner lays hands upon a client's body (commonly over clothing, which differs from massage therapy) in order to direct the flow of Reiki to specific areas of the client's body and more generally, to their energy field.

However, physical touch is not always necessary, as some clients dislike touch for various reasons, and some practitioners like to "hover" a few inches over the body to perceive energy. As your own practice will highlight, energy does not need touch to flow or be felt. This is one of the reasons why distance Reiki works as well as an in-person session; for those of you familiar with an intuitive reading, it's similar in that it's about tuning into a client's energy, but distance Reiki focuses on assessing your energetic well-being (perceived as "flow" or lack thereof) rather than on answering a question you'd have for a reading, for example.

Reiki energy flows through our bodies like water. We're born with breath, water, and life force (rei) in our bodies; we're animated by and produce energy (ki). It's then a choice whether we breathe deeply, whether the water flows within us as we hydrate, and whether the universal life force of Reiki, evolves from a trickle to a strong, steady stream.

This state of alignment helps you create ideal overall health of mind, heart, and body. This holistic practice allows universal life force energy to flow freely through your body to help your physical, emotional, and mind bodies to do what they naturally know how to do: restore and heal.

MEDITATION & RELAXATION

In legal and practical terms, Reiki is considered a meditation and relaxation technique, which can be assisted by a professional Reiki practitioner in the formal setting of a scheduled session.

Again from a legal perspective, words such as "healing" are generally avoided when describing Reiki, because they often get misconstrued as cure claims. Throughout this book, variations of the word "healing" are used to refer to the process or cultivating and returning to a state of wellness (homeostasis) and a lifestyle of harmony, via healthy habits and life-honouring practices personal to each and everyone.

Health and wellness are complex systems that reflect the people who embody them; health and wellness are in constant motion, and result from a number of practices and treatments, depending on the person and their unique situation. In this way, as an alternative health practice, and in a supportive role, Reiki fosters healing.

To be clear, my belief and experience with Reiki is not exclusive of allopathic medicine and psychological treatment. I do not discourage seeking appropriate medical and mental health help for any issue you may be experiencing. Healing is a complex process of layers, physical, mental, emotional and spiritual, and one should give themselves the best chances of recovery by reaching for and accepting relevant help that also feels aligned with their values.

In fact, no traditional or alternative health care practitioner should ever discourage you from getting adequate and well-rounded health and wellness treatment and support you feel might help you. As an example, when I suffered from hypothyroidism, I accepted the hormonal support I was prescribed, while I continued to work on the areas of my life that contributed to the imbalance.

I also know from both my studies and first-hand experience that touch (whether your own or that of a trusted practitioner) will shift the body's nervous system into the parasympathetic mode, or what we call the "rest and digest" or even "tend and befriend." It is the only state in which we can cultivate physical health, as it allows our body to restore, properly function, eliminate toxins and stress hormones created in the sympathetic state, or what we all know as "fight, flight, or freeze."

From experience, I've seen the immediate and tangible shift in my students' and clients' demeanour when they shift into their parasympathetic mode. They shift into this parasympathetic mode through various methods, from breathing deeply and mindfully, meditating, or in light of this guide, by practising Reiki yoga. Their heart rate slows, their breath deepens, and their bodies visibly relax. I can see their faces soften and their postures opening as they return to a natural stance, less defensive or aggressive. Of course, their mood lifts, or there's an emotional release, and their mood (energy) changes—all that in a few brief moments! It is certainly empowering to participate in one's own healing process.

However you choose to approach Reiki, it is a holistic practice that needs to be experienced first-hand to be integrated. Reiki as a lifestyle contributes to overall wellness.

REIKI PRINCIPLES & DAILY AFFIRMATION

There are Reiki principles that have been formulated as a daily affirmation or prayer, to remind us of the lifestyle Reiki fosters. Reiki is not a religious practice, but rather a spiritual one like meditation. These affirmations are considered daily practices because they require mindfulness and renewal of our commitment. Whether you are an avid practitioner of Reiki, or a new Reiki yoga practitioner on your own journey, these are simple and healthy principles to keep front of mind.

TRADITIONAL REIKI PRINCIPLES

Just for today, I will not worry.
Just for today, I will not anger.
Just for today, I will be grateful.
Just for today, I will do my work honestly.
Just for today, I will be kind to every living being.

Though I understand the sentiment in the traditional version above, I prefer my personal version, which taps into the law of attraction and neuro-linguistic programming principles of manifestation, empowerment, and shaping our external reality. I also learned from an indigenous Elder that simplified language of action in the present tense is always more powerful and effective.

Phrases such as "I am [name the feeling / role]" and "I choose [name the feeling / calling / action / situation you are inviting in as few words as possible]" are potent manifesting tools. Don't add "to do" or "to have" or "to be" between your choosing and the object of your choice. Instead of saying, "I choose to practise Reiki yoga," you could simply say "I choose Reiki yoga" and allow it to unfold into your life in the appropriate manner best suited to you. These principles apply to all affirmations practice. **Any affirmations you choose to adopt are more powerful in simplified, present-tense language; remember that "I am" and "I choose" are your go-to formulas.**

With this wisdom in my heart centre, this is my take on the Reiki principles.

BRIGHT STAR WOMAN REIKI PRINCIPLES

Today, I choose acceptance/peace.
Today, I choose peace/forgiveness.
Today, I choose gratitude/contentment/joy.
Today, I choose integrity/honesty/alignment.
Today, I choose kindness/love/respect.

Choose the words that resonate with you. For instance, if you feel acceptance better conveys the opposite of worry to you, then use that word. If peace better conveys the opposite of anger to you, then use it. I put options in each of those statements above to invoke the sentiments of the traditional Reiki principles, but I go with how I feel in the moment.

ATTUNEMENTS

I have received numerous questions about the significance of attunements, and questions regarding whether they were necessary to practise Reiki yoga.

Attunements are initiation ceremonies in which aspiring Reiki practitioners receive symbols, above their bodies and into their hands, in order to be introduced to the energy of Reiki and become its channels.

Attunement ceremonies are powerful experiences where one can discover energy in a new way, especially if they have never received Reiki or other energy-healing modalities, such as reflexology, EFT Tapping, Trager, or shamanic practices for example.

Usually, attunements are performed by Reiki master teachers and are accompanied by training or workshops to give context to the energy and its use as a wellness modality. In the Usui lineage, they are generally offered in three or four levels. Level one is the apprentice, level two is the practitioner, level three is the master (or the professional, which is the one thing most schools of thought agree on), and in some schools of thought, level 4 is the master teacher.

As a rule, levels one and two don't generally charge for their service as a profession. Though there is some debate, usually level threes are considered professionals, and occasionally, some consider them teachers as well. One of my teachers taught me that level one was a student, level two was a qualified professional and level three was a master and a teacher. Yet, another teacher taught me that levels one and two are students, but the level twos were encouraged to offer Reiki as a secondary modality to their profession (as in the case of body workers) or as a volunteer. According to that teacher, only level threes (masters in all schools of thought) could actually be considered professional Reiki practitioners. That same teacher also encouraged the four-level teaching system, distinguishing master practitioners from master teachers; because as she put it "not all practitioners feel called to teach and train others."

It is my personal and professional view, that without attunements, Reiki can be experienced as a receiver (which is also the belief of established Reiki practitioners), but also as a self-practitioner. This is the part that seems ground-breaking and for which I have received criticism. Traditional practitioners do no believe that non-attuned self-practitioners can "actually channel Reiki." I personally believe this to be archaic and limited 3D thinking that forgets that Reiki's own nature is energy and that it cannot be contained by one's initiation or training level.

Much in the same way as music can be taught, it is also felt and experienced, and it can be created as well as appreciated without training. Will one's ability to understand and create music improve with training? Absolutely. Yet it is not necessary to get started, should training not be available or of use for the person's own journey. Not everyone needs to be a concert pianist to love the piano, while one can still learn and love it, whether they are self-taught or take years of lessons.

I know energy to be everywhere and accessible to anyone willing to connect with integrity. Reiki doesn't just appear because I drew symbols on your hands; the idea is that those symbols open you up as a channel. However, the energy was always there to be harnessed and shared.

Yes, I am personally an initiate because I am now a Reiki master teacher in at least two Reiki modalities (Usui and Blue Star) and continue to learn all the time. I have begun my initiation in Karuna Reiki®. That said, I have seen firsthand, non-initiates channel Reiki in self-practice, and I've seen this in both children and adults. This book is based on this observation and this belief that anyone can channel Reiki, and even more successfully with coaching, experience and yes, formal learning as well.

I see non-initiate Reiki self-practitioners as similar to yoga practitioners who have never attended group yoga classes and never pursued yoga teacher training; they can practice, but their knowledge and experience is somewhat limited, and hence, they should definitely not teach others. But these "non-iniates" (or self-taught practitioners) could blossom with appropriate encouragement and formal learning.

I have had beautiful experiences in my own attunements and was in awe of the shifts that I witness when attuning my clients. I encourage dedicated (self-)practitioners to seek attunements, whether with me through my website (brightstarwoman.com), a local Reiki master teacher, or any Reiki master teacher that feels like a great match for them.

The challenge in pursuing a Reiki attunement is that Reiki is still a largely unregulated field of practice and there are almost as many styles and approaches as there are teachers. There are professional associations, but they are not regulating bodies. At the time of writing this book, despite having over sixteen years of experience with Reiki, I still do not belong to a professional Reiki association. Perhaps I will one day, but I have not yet felt the need to apply to one. I am however, an accredited professional of different modalities with the Complementary Therapists Accredited Association (CTAA).

The takeaway with attunements is that I encourage you to experience at least a level one with a trusted Reiki master teacher, but if resources near you aren't what you would hope, or if you are waiting to see if you want to invest in taking one (usually the most affordable level, around a few hundred dollars) don't let that stop you from learning Reiki yoga now.

Should you want to explore Reiki further, whether personally or professionally, I would urge you to complete all other levels of your chosen Reiki lineage (i.e., Usui, Blue Star, Karuna Reiki®, etc.) before offering Reiki professionally and asking for compensation (more on that in The Ethics of Sharing Reiki Yoga). This book is not a replacement for an attunement, but rather an introduction to a hybrid practice, which can only be enhanced by Reiki attunements and yoga classes. Even if you only seek Reiki training for your own practice, it will amplify your experience of Reiki itself, as well as deepen your own practice of Reiki yoga.

WHAT IS YOGA?

THOUGH IT IS ROOTED in philosophy (documented in the yoga sutras), yoga is an ancient Indian practice of breath (pranayama), postures (asanas), and guiding principles (yamas and niyamas) to facilitate meditation and foster the harmony of body and mind. Ultimately, the practice of yoga aims to lead the yogi(ni) to enlightenment: knowing of the Self, the Divine, and the Universe.

The word "yoga" translates into "union" as well as "discipline," thus it is the practice of joining body and mind, as well as cultivating our union with our personal sense of the divine or universe; it is a tool for the blossoming of our own spirituality.

Patanjali, the author of the Yoga Sutras, has classified yoga practice into eight limbs. They are defined as yama (abstinences), niyama (observances), asana (postures), pranayama (breathing), pratyahara (withdrawal), dharana (concentration), dhyana (meditation), and samadhi (union, integration). Modern (or westernized) yoga often eclipses at least six limbs by focusing on asanas, or the physical practice of postures, and pranayama, the breathing techniques. These eight limbs of yoga are meant to guide our lifestyle to foster harmony within ourselves and with others, overall health, and spiritual unity.

Yoga is a product of the culture and time that birthed it; it is rich with polytheistic mythos to explain how the practice was discovered and evolved. That said, it is essentially a secular practice open to all.

Naturally, there are wonderful physical and mental health benefits to having a regular yoga practice, which may include asanas, breathwork, chanting, and meditation. The benefits, which include fitness and flexibility to stress reduction, mental clarity, and increased happiness, have been observed and published through many studies. It was also demonstrated that a yoga practice helps curb anxiety and alleviate depression.

COMBINING REIKI & YOGA

BOTH OF THESE ancient methods share fundamental philosophical principles. Reiki is founded on the idea that our body has layers of energy and circulates through currents (channels); yoga teaches that the body has koshas (i.e., 5 layers of energy) and that *prana* (i.e., life energy) circulates through the body through *nadis* (i.e., energy streams) and concentrate around *chakras* (i.e., energy centres). Upon reflection, one realizes that ki and prana are different words to express energy, with the exception that "ki" (or "chi" with the Chinese) can also refer to disembodied energy, like in the case of feng shui (the art of the harmonious living space). Prana is believed to only inhabit living creatures.

Reiki and yoga are both eastern health practices that rely on the mind-body connection. They both also foster the development of one's personal spiritual practice and holistic view of the body and health, shifting toward the concept of wellness. Through the independent practice of these disciplines, it becomes obvious combining these two complementary practices creates a powerhouse of self-healing.

THE BENEFITS OF PRACTISING REIKI YOGA

STUDIES HAVE DEMONSTRATED that the regular practice of yoga aids in creating overall health. Yoga improves breathing and increases vitality, it reduces anxiety and helps with stress management. Yoga improves flexibility and builds strength and muscle tone, and assists circulatory health and metabolic function. This means it also helps manage blood pressure and maintain a healthy weight. Body awareness, which the practice of yoga fosters, is also crucial in athletic performance, but its great appeal as we age is that it helps prevent injury. In recent years, studies have found that yoga alleviates the symptoms of depression, and even assists in reversing the DNA damage that causes this mental illness.

There are significantly less studies to support the claims that Reiki is an effective holistic healing approach. Reiki practitioners will tell you that this modality aids relaxation, assists in the body's natural healing processes, and a return to homeostasis (i.e., the body's state of optimal function). Practising and receiving reiki develops emotional, mental, and spiritual well-being. In legal terms, it is generally recognized as a traditional Japanese healing art, which is alleged to assist in relaxation through the channeling of healing energy, and fosters the conditions to induce deep relaxation, help people cope with personal and physical difficulties, relieve emotional stress, and improve overall wellness.

What is known, however, is that a person who allows themselves to relax, and engages in practices that help shift their nervous system from the sympathetic (fight, flight, or freeze responses) to the parasympathetic (tend and befriend, rest and digest responses) will generally report lower stress levels, cultivate a positive outlook, and show a healthier immune system. Moreover, a person who has a well-established self-care and/or a wellness routine will report greater confidence and satisfaction.

Meditation, which is an aspect of the Reiki yoga practice, has a well-documented list of physical, mental and emotional health benefits. Of the long list recognized by the allopathic medical community, regular meditation practice was shown to physically decrease blood pressure, improve sleep, reduce inflammation and chronic pain, assist in releasing addictions, and assist in reducing age-related memory loss. Studies have shown that meditation improves mental and emotional health, namely by reducing stress, alleviating chronic anxiety, alleviating depression, increasing the ability to focus, and to develop self-awareness. Regular meditation supports kindness and compassionate behaviour, which in turn promotes healthier, happier, more fulfilling relationships.

Reiki yoga as a hybrid practice offers all of these individual disciplines combined benefits, as well as developing a greater awareness and sense of self. Practising Reiki yoga also fosters the creation and maintenance of a meditation practice, helps to develop a stronger intuition and build trust, and supports the creation and respect of healthy boundaries in all areas of life. Reiki yoga is a holistic wellness practice.

REIKI & THERAPEUTIC TOUCH: THE SOMATIC EFFECT

Many beginners and non-Reiki practitioners often ask me if it's normal that they "don't feel anything" or "don't feel what they think they're supposed to feel." They'll even ask me: "Is it even working if I can't feel anything / don't feel any different / don't believe in this stuff?"

My resounding answer is always: "Trust the process, and trust that you are getting exactly what you need from this."

Studies have shown that touch is not only highly personal, but depending on context, it can also be therapeutic. Moreover, our own touch is healing because it brings us back to ourselves, in presence, in self-care and in compassion. Therapeutic touch is linked to stress reduction and a shift in the nervous system (from the sympathetic "fight, flight, or freeze" to the parasympathetic "rest and digest / tend and befriend"). This is one of the ways massage therapy benefits the body-mind connection and overall wellness.

In an article published on October 20, 2016 by Noel Wight titled *"Touch Transforms Lives"*, the Somatic Therapy Center (thesomatictherapycenter.com) published the following statement on their website, which resumes the somatic effect of touch on overall wellness and healing:

To the extent that the absence of touch is deleterious, the presence of touch can be equally as beneficial and even transformative.

Touch is experienced as a physical sensation and also affectively as an emotion. Touch communicates feelings. It soothes and signals safety and trust. A warm nurturing touch slows the heat rate and calms cardiovascular stress. Studies have shown that hugging produces oxytocin, the "love hormone," that reduces stress, lowers cortisol levels and increases a sense of trust and security. Touch also conveys compassion and opens our hearts. We say we are "touched" when we are moved emotionally by an experience. There is also a need for psychological touch – attention, care, recognition, love, – that is as great as the need for physical touch.

As we understand the effects of lack of touch and recognize the benefits of touch, it becomes clear that therapies that use direct touch can have a depth and potency that can access healing that is not available without it.

Touch is the key that gives us access to the body's knowings. Our bodies are memory holders. It is in and through our five senses that we live our lives. Our bodies remember and are shaped by the events, feelings, and thoughts that we have experienced. It has been our constant companion and as such carries a record of our lives in its every cell. Touch is a direct doorway to this storehouse of knowledge.

People often think of psychological issues as taking place in the mind, however, over the past 30 years of seeing clients we know, and science has now confirmed, that there is no separation of body and mind; they are inseparable. Feelings take place in the body as well as the mind. The body is the vehicle for emotional expression and that happens primarily through movement. Sometimes the feeling can be expressed through a sad facial expression, an angry hand movement, a stomped foot or large jump for joy. There are also the chemical shifts in the body that are associated with emotions. Candace Pert in her research actually identified the molecule of emotion. Touch can access these emotions far more readily than talk alone. Touch that is accompanied by the compassionate dialogue of awareness promotes both physical and emotional healing.

Although the above quote pertains specifically to somatic therapy as a field of care, it clearly describes the benefits of touch in therapeutic approaches.

Furthermore, our own therapeutic touch, one that is gentle, kind, and attentive to our own needs, acts on the somatic level to communicate a sense of safety, ease and self-compassion. The body interprets therapeutic touch as care and support, and is able to release tension and emotions that may have been lodged in the body's organs (as believed in Traditional Chinese Medicine) and/or in its energy field (as believed in yoga and Reiki practice). In short, touch makes us feel safe and held.

The truth is, energy will flow in our body, consciously or unconsciously. We can develop an awareness of this flow, and of energy in general, with practice. When you drink a cup of water, do you have to think about absorbing it or does your body just do it? Of course, you can drink mindfully, making the experience meditative in nature and increasing its potency by raising yours and your body's awareness of the drink of water. Feeling the water on your tongue and cheeks, noticing its temperature, tasting the liquid, swallowing it intentionally and feeling it coat your throat, sliding down your esophagus and landing in the belly. That said, whether you think about it or not, your body will receive and process the water.

Energy is similar; you can approach it mindfully, or not. You can be affected unconsciously by the energies of others, of your environment, of your chosen nourishment (food, drink, and other consumables like art forms and hobbies, such as the music to which you listen or the books you choose to read). Or, you can choose to be more intentional about the energies you welcome and encourage into your inner sanctum and your daily life.

ENERGY AWARENESS & THE SENSES

An important component of the practice of Reiki yoga is developing our own energy awareness, and that of the universal life force energy as it flows through us. You can certainly foster your awareness of energy (your own and that of others) through practice. These practices can absolutely be Reiki yoga, but they can be anything that you do mindfully, as the observer of your own self and your own behaviour.

When you practise yoga and meditation, when you colour or express yourself artfully, when you listen to an inspiring piece of music, when you are drawn into a story or film and feel engaged, when you express yourself creatively, dance or laugh with abandonment to just BE. All of these are ways we can ground ourselves into our bodies, into the present, which is truly the only moment of power. The present is when we are most ourselves, most creative, most intuitive, and at our most powerful. When we are present, we can observe, listen, feel, taste, smell. And then our other extra-sensory perception awakens because we've created space for these senses to be tuned.

Just as we have stronger physical senses, as we develop our energy awareness, our intuitive self may have strengths and manifest itself in specific ways.

In a meditation practice, we often anchor ourselves in the breath: observing it, feeling it, visualizing with it, listening to it, and so on. The five physical senses are also used as tools to anchor ourselves into our bodies and in the present moment. As we use these senses, we refine them and we may notice that one of them is stronger, or easier to tap into. Our extra-sensory perception works in a similar way.

When we practise Reiki yoga, we are learning to notice energy by using our senses AND extra-sensory perception, because there is more than just what is happening in our physical bodies, though that's certainly a part of it! As we tune-in and scan our bodies, we are also scanning our energy field. In this process, we are prompted to notice sensations, feelings, thoughts, images, temperature, tastes, words, areas of the body that "pop up," or that may draw more attention, or do so persistently. Though there are certain guidelines, or methods that yield results more consistently, there's no way to "scan incorrectly." Moreover, whatever way *you* perceive the messages from your body and energy field is right for you. With practice, you will notice that your perceptions will come to you more easily in one form (or a few).

For traditional Reiki practitioners, it was said that heat (or broadly, temperature) indicated the flow of energy. This is only a small portion of how energy can be perceived! So take heart, if you're a "cold handed healer," it doesn't mean that Reiki doesn't flow, that "you have no innate skill," or that your Reiki yoga practice isn't working; just pay attention to the ways in which you ARE receiving messages, intuitive guidance. Notice how Reiki is benefiting YOU, both during and after your practice.

If you're skeptical or tempted to give in to worry, keep a journal with your experiences and how you felt in your body, mind, and mood, after practising Reiki yoga (this can be a useful practitioner record of your client experiences as well). You can review it and notice trends. A life coach once told me: "You can tone down the voice of doubt under the weight of your evidence list." This is a list you can draw up of your accomplishments and blessings. Essentially, it's a list of all the ways in which you are succeeding at your projects, goals, and aspirations. This evidence list helps you celebrate on the journey (experience and process oriented), and not just when you have achieved a goal (results oriented). This principle applies here in the form of your recorded experience, such as journaling your practice.

WHO CAN PRACTISE REIKI YOGA?

THOUGH IT MAY APPEAR to be overgeneralising to say that everyone can benefit from this hybrid practice, it is true. Individually, yoga and Reiki are modalities that benefit any and everyone physically, mentally and emotionally. They are both established self-care practices. Beginners, experienced yogi(ni)s and Reiki practitioners alike will discover nuggets of wellness from this hybrid practice.

That being said, there are perhaps less obvious "ideal candidates" for the Reiki yoga practice.

- People who are less physically fit or have mobility limitations may prefer this gentle style as most poses can be adapted or swapped for a milder more accessible version.
- People who are interested in a physical or tactile meditation will appreciate this introspective, yet subtly

physical approach to meditation (i.e., kinesthetic learners will appreciate this approach to energy).
- People who suffer from chronic physical and mental conditions will benefit from the body slowing down and reconnecting with the breath and energy.
- People who suffer from anxiety or depression will benefit from the gentle present-moment anchoring of Reiki yoga.
- People who want to develop their intuition, build self-confidence and trust in the Universe/Spirit/Creator/God and create and maintain healthy boundaries, will benefit from this (self-) awareness practice.

Anyone with chronic physical or mental conditions can benefit from tuning into their body, slowing down, breathing intentionally, and calming the nervous system, listening to the body's messages, and this is what Reiki yoga enables. Offering gentle Reiki energy where needed, helps the body to soften into peace and release energetic debris at one's own pace.

If you suffer from anxiety (unhealthy future projection), or from depression (unhealthy past projection), Reiki yoga anchors you in the present and reminds you that you are enough, worthy, and you have absolutely all you need within.

Reiki yoga cultivates self-care and intuition, which are both superpowers in our fast-paced, productivity-focused world. If you want to develop your intuition, Reiki yoga is an ideal practice of self-awareness and trust. It also fosters healthier relationships as it helps us notice our values and limits, helping us kindly reinforce those boundaries in all areas of our lives. Reiki yoga reminds us how powerful we are when we are BE-ing.

Reiki yoga can help support your various situations and help you grow...

Reiki yoga beneficial on many levels

BODY	MIND	HEART & SOUL	LIFE TRANSITIONS
• Chronic pain • Chronic conditions • Injury & recovery • Sleep issues • Digestive issues • Hormonal imbalances • Develop body awareness, create healthy habits	• Anxiety • Depression • Stress management • Develop a meditation practice • Develop self-awareness, create boundaries	• Burnout • Recovery programs (PTSD, Substance abuse, behavioural) • Boundary setting • Creating healthful habits • Develop your intuition, build trust	• Life transitions • Career transitions • Moving homes • Relationship changes, such as separation/divorce • Grief & loss • Develop perspective, find peace

MOST SUITABLE YOGA STYLES

BASED on the plethora of yoga styles now studied and taught all over the world, one could easily argue that Reiki can be practised with any style of yoga, and this would be technically correct. In fact, I encourage you to try for yourself different yoga practices with your Reiki practice to see what works for you.

Although Reiki has a therapeutic approach, it can be used to boost energy, as well as restore. The style of yoga practised will determine the perspective or goal in mind; a hatha or flow practice will be more vigorous than a yin or restorative practice, which of course, will have a different impact on the muscles, connective tissues, organs, and energy expended and produced.

That being said, there are a few styles of yoga that lend themselves well, or more easily, to both the introspective aspect of connecting with Reiki universal life force energy, as well as practising a self-treatment of Reiki. I've found my students to be most receptive to gentle hatha and flow, yin and restorative yoga.

When you need more grounding and integration, yin and restorative are the go-to choices, as the practice is on the floor, slow, low-impact (physically), and introspective.

When you need an energy boost and to break out of a rut, gentle hatha and flow are the preferred practices, as there is more movement, the body is more directly involved in the renewal of energy, and the practice resembles an active meditation. I personally don't gravitate toward or share many (if any at all) standing poses in a gentle hatha or flow Reiki yoga class. We can flow close to the ground to stay deeply rooted and present, which is also an important component of the Reiki practice.

A vinyasa or power Reiki practice is possible, but I wouldn't recommend it for beginners of Reiki yoga; it requires an established yoga practice as well as an established Reiki yoga practice. Holding or moving through challenging poses and sequences requires a lot of energy and focus, and a yogi would need to remember the intention of Reiki and self-treatment, and that means getting creative in finding the hand positions, visualizations and symbols, and chants to focus the Reiki energy at key moments.

HANDS: HEALING PORTALS

THOUGH REIKI IS its own healing art, I wanted to highlight how many cultures have recognized and fostered the existence of energy and have practised healing using the hands as their vehicle. Our bodies are complex, beautiful, and miraculous! I believe our hands hold magic...

MUDRAS

The yogic tradition has practised mudras (translated to both "seal" and "gesture"), by forming shapes with the hands and creating light pressure on different points, which in turn stimulate certain parts of the brain, by which messages are communicated to the body, creating physical, mental, and emotional effects. Moreover, we now know that changes on those levels also mean broader energetic changes, and vice versa. Mudras are commonly called "the yoga of the hands." Mudras aren't as well understood (or practised) in the Western world as asanas (yoga poses), but this is changing as we are discovering the quiet strength and subtle medicine of mudras. We can practise them for as little as a few breaths to several minutes, and repeat this practice several times a day to foster qualities we wish to experience (physically, mentally, emotionally, spiritually). Other than the classic chin/gyan (for wisdom) and anjali (for balance and dedication) mudras, my favourite mudras include kalesvara (the Master of Time), trimurti (for life transitions), vajrapradama (unshakable trust), abhaya hridaya (fearless heart).

MERIDIANS AND REFLEXOLOGY

In Traditional Chinese Medicine (TCM), the theory of meridian lines has guided the development of reflexology, acupuncture, shiatsu, and similar disciplines. As a certified hand reflexologist, I find this method especially fascinating as it is so portable. Our bodies are mapped out in our hands; both hands forming a whole picture of the physical body. I've witnesses this time and again with clients. Even my husband, who is a cerebral, analytical person, was surprised and amazed that I could identify with precision his physical ailments by what I perceived in his hands during a reflexology treatment I gave him.

Reflexology also claims that by massaging the feet for two minutes, we activate the lower meridians (kidney/bladder, liver/gallbladder, stomach/spleen) and by massage the hands for two minutes (each), we stimulate upper meridians (stomach/spleen, heart/intestines, lungs/colon). And this is true without sophisticated knowledge of meridian lines, zones, or pressure points!

Professional EFT (Emotional Freedom Technique) practitioners will tell you that there are several tapping points in the hands, including the karate chop point, situated on the side of the hand, where most set-up statements are made in this healing modality. There are also points near the fingertips and between knuckles. Though I am not an expert in the history of Tapping it is the Emotional Freedom Technique created by Dr Roger Callahan as Thought Field Therapy (or Tapping Therapy) who founded the tapping on Meridian Theory, as described by Traditional Chinese Medicine. Tapping Therapy was further developed by Gary Craig, a Master of neuro-linguistic programming (NLP) to bring powerful phrasing to this technique that already utilized the mind-body connection and meridians. EFT Tapping helps voice the emotions that may be otherwise trapped in the body, release them with acceptance, and reframe our experience in a constructive, self-honouring light.

In indigenous communities, Shamans and Elders also avoid "pointing" as they understand that powerful energy is directed from our hands and fingers.

Hands are more than practical body parts and everyday tools; they are truly healing portals.

PART 1 HIGHLIGHTS

- Reiki yoga is a hybrid practice that combines the Indian wellness practice of yoga and the Japanese healing art of Reiki.
- Reiki yoga is a therapeutic practice that uses energy (through touch and sensing when we scan the energy field for example, through movement, breath, visualization, and sound) to nurture presence and self-awareness, and foster a state of homeostasis to enable healing.
- Because it is energy, Reiki can be channeled for self-practice without an attunement, but should not be practised on others without receiving an attunement from a Reiki master teacher. Pursuing at least a level one in Reiki is encouraged for personal practice, if nothing else, but is not required to use this book.
- Reiki yoga can be practised with any form of traditional yoga. However, therapeutic styles, such as gentle hatha

and flow, yin, and restorative yoga may be a more organic pairing, depending on what the practitioner needs.
- Energy awareness can take on many forms, namely through the sense, and each person's experience is unique and valid.
- Reiki yoga can benefit anyone on the physical, emotional, mental, and spiritual levels.
- Reiki yoga helps develop presence, mindfulness, intuition, and trust.
- Reiki yoga supports healthy lifestyle choices and relationships through self-respect and boundary setting.
- Reiki yoga supports other wellness practices.
- Hands are considered healing portals in many cultures and traditions.

Part two

Shape Your Practice

STRUCTURING YOUR REIKI YOGA PRACTICE
GROUNDING & INTENTION

THIS IS a common practice in all yoga classes; take the time to arrive and centre yourself with deep, mindful, equal breaths. Perhaps you count to four on both the inhales and exhales. With your inner gaze, scan your body head to toe, with the intention to observe, not judge. Notice your energy, mood, thoughts, and particular sensations living in your body.

From this place of awareness, choose an intention for your practice; the intention is the theme in which you choose to move and breathe, and maybe it is something you wish to cultivate, invite, or even send to someone.

For example, your theme can be compassion. You can offer yourself more compassion especially in poses and through movements that you find challenging, or where you sense frustration. You may choose to cultivate harmony, or to invite abundance, or even simply to send love to someone you wish to support. When it comes to setting an intention, choose what speaks to you in the moment.

As you begin, if you are seated for the grounding portion of your practice, I recommend opening with your hands in anjali mudra (i.e., together in a prayer over your heart) and a chant, such as Om, to set the tone and open your sacred space. Beyond the use of sound (voice, bells, drum, rattles, etc.), spaces can also be cleared of negativity and stagnant energy, as well as be harmonized by using herbal medicines, such as sage smudge (i.e., sacred smoke) or herbal and floral spray (i.e., in an essential oil spray).

If you choose to ground yourself by lying on your back in savasana, you can still open with a chant, but the anjali mudra (i.e., salutation mudra, balancing mind and body) becomes a bit more challenging. Simply rest on your back and chant Om (or another mantra of your choice) if it feels right. Notice the experience of the sound vibrating through your body from the ground (as opposed to sitting). You will likely feel it reverberating differently.

If you are a teacher leading a Reiki yoga class, you may choose to chant on behalf of your class, if they aren't comfortable chanting yet or if you feel they can benefit from receiving sound, rather than producing it.

REIKI ACTIVATION

THE PROCESS of Reiki activation is specific to Reiki practice and by extension, to Reiki yoga. It's the mindful invitation and fostering the flow of Reiki energy into your body.

Reiki activation is a little bit like plugging in your laptop; it functions on battery, but it'll use source energy if it's plugged into an electric outlet.

I most often use a guided visualisation of both the inner fire and the universal flow of energy and invite it into my body (meditation below).

You can also simply repeat the mantra (in your mind or out loud, three times) "Reiki," which can also be combined with rubbing your hands together to create heat and call the energy into your hands (the channel's output).

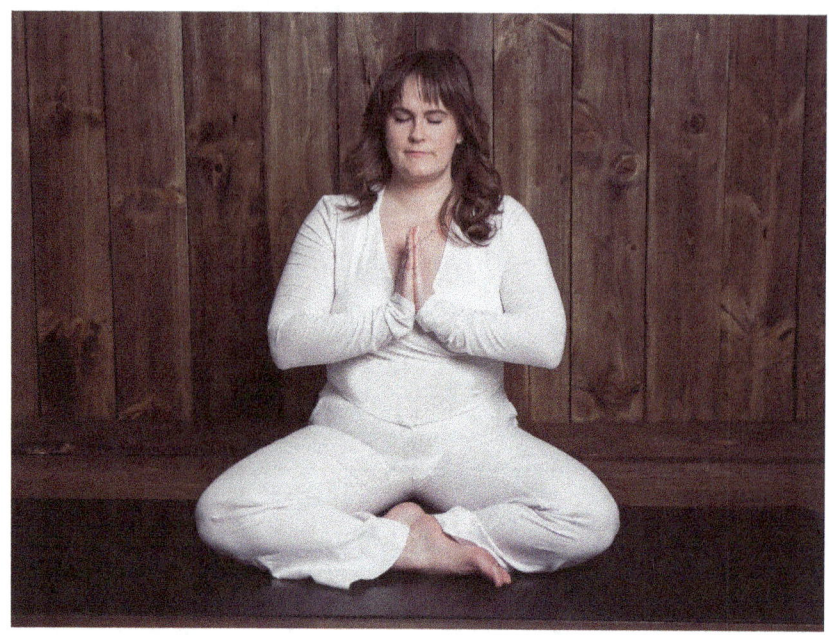

In a comfortable seat, hands together, activate the flow of Reiki through visualization. You can also do this lying down, arms by your side.

A Reiki practitioner also knows to invite the Reiki guides in opening a sacred space for the practice; I encourage you to invite your Reiki guides (in your mind or out loud) in creating this healing space for you.

Another suggestion would be to chant Om Reiki Reiki Reiki Om at this point, especially if the grounding happened in savasana (lying down on your back).

Go to BrightStarWoman.com to grab your free Reiki meditation, which serves as a wonderful Reiki activation for your practice.

SCANNING YOUR BODY & ENERGY FIELD

BEFORE BEGINNING ANY REIKI TREATMENT, a practitioner scans the client's body with their hands (where the Reiki concentrates) to get a feel for what's going on in that person's energy field. It is also true when doing a self-treatment. This means that if you're practising Reiki yoga, you'll want to scan yourself as a way of tuning into your body (or rather, bodies, as we consider the emotional, mental, and spiritual as part of our whole selves). Reiki scanning of the aura becomes easier with practice. You may begin to sense changes in temperature, tingling or specific sensations, see images in your mind's eye, or get a thought or feeling when you hover over a certain part of your own body.

SELF-TREATMENT

THIS IS when you get creative! There are traditional hand positions that are recommended to get an overall treatment, and then, you can add your own. I personally treat head to toe, even on myself, unless I'm having an emotional day, or feel uprooted and disconnected, in which case I treat my heart first (centre of all seven chakras) and then go head to toe. Ensure your hands are slightly cupped to focus the energy into your hands. A useful image to remember the cupping is that of trying to drink water with your hands; holding flowing water is easier to collect in your palms when your hands form a recipient, than if your fingers are spread and palms are flat...

You can approach the self-treatment from the physical body, from the chakras' energy centres perspective, or both. I tend to combine traditional Usui Reiki hand positions with non-traditional, following chakra locations and intuitive guidance of where I feel my hands are calling me.

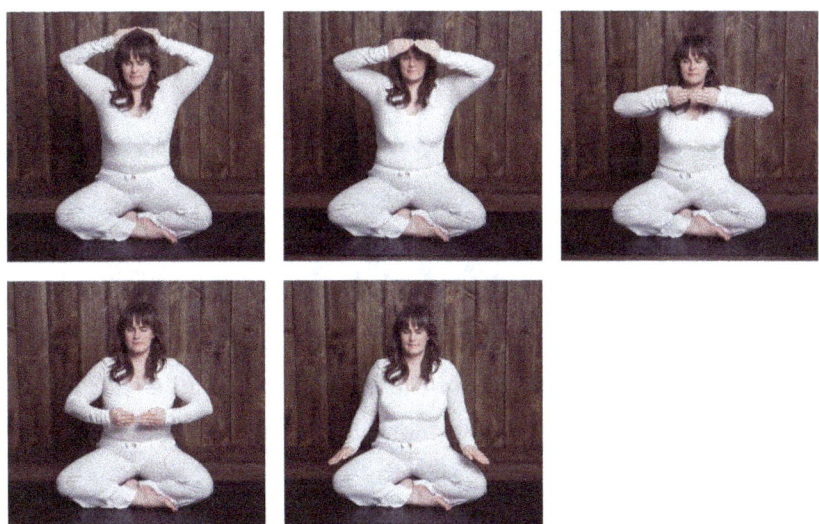

Eyes closed, scan your energy feel by floating your hands a few inches (centimeters) above your body.

Below, are examples of hand positions for self-treatment.

HAND POSITIONS

Consider the hand positions included here a mix of traditional Usui and contemporary (or "intuitive") hand positions to facilitate your self-treatment. When practising Reiki on yourself, whether simply in Reiki practice or in Reiki yoga practice, always gently cup your hands (i.e., concave palm, fingers pressed together, like drinking water from your hand) to allow for the energy to "pool" and focus from your hand to the area of treatment.

HEAD

There are several hand positions to practise on and around your head when giving a self-treatment.

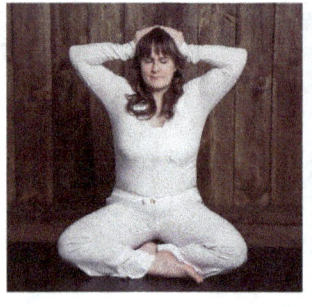 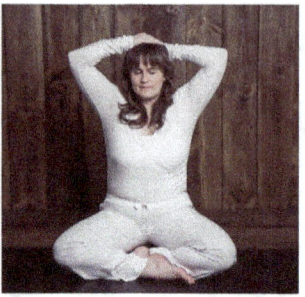

Above: place your hands upon the top of your head either one in front of the other (i.e., palm to palm, fingers in opposite direction) or side by side (i.e., finger tips touching). *Chakra: Crown*

Forehead + occiput: place one hand on your forehead and the other behind your head, at the base of your skull, like you are holding your own head and sending Reiki white light between your palms. *Chakra: Third Eye*

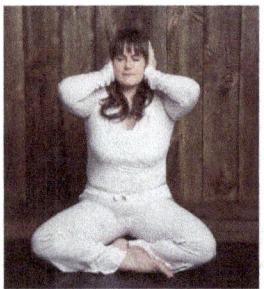 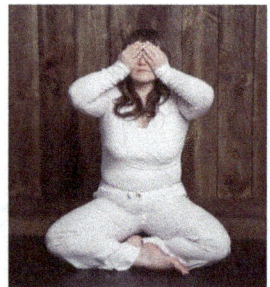 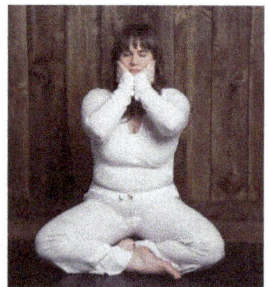

Ears: place your hands on each ear like you are holding headphones, tuning out the noise. *Chakra: Throat.*

Eyes: place your hands over your eyes, allowing finger tips to rest between the eyebrows. *Chakra: Third Eye.*

Jaw, mouth: place your hands on either side of your jaw, then place your hand(s) over your mouth. *Chakra: Throat.*

NECK

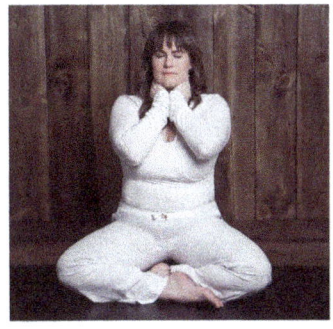

Throat: place both hands on your throat (palm to palm, fingers pointing to the neck), of float your hands if more comfortable. *Chakra: Throat.*

Neck: place one or both hands on the neck (do not interlace fingers), finger tips may touch, or you can place one hand over the other to "support" your neck. *Chakra: Throat.*

SHOULDERS AND ARMS

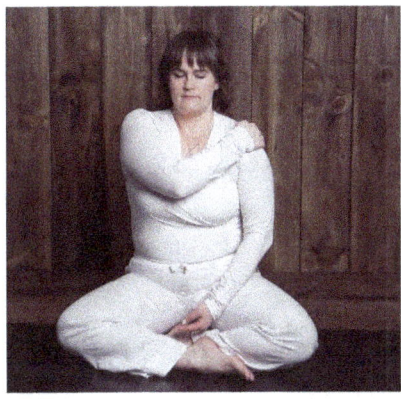 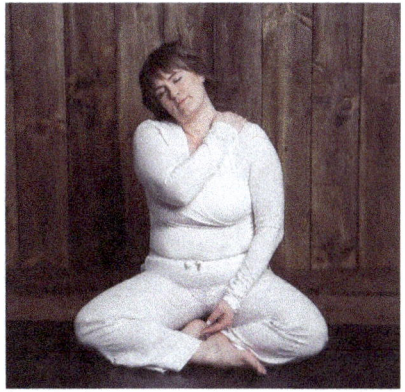

Shoulder and trapeze muscle: lean your head to the right side, place your right hand on your left trapeze. Bring your head back to neutral, move your hand to your shoulder and work your way down the arm: upper arm, elbow, forearm, wrist, then palm to palm. *Chakras: Throat, Heart.*

Do the other arm.

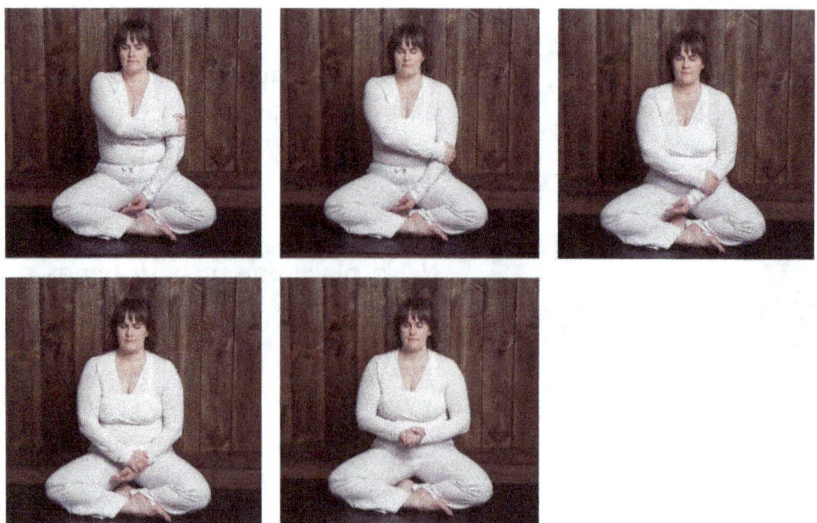

TORSO

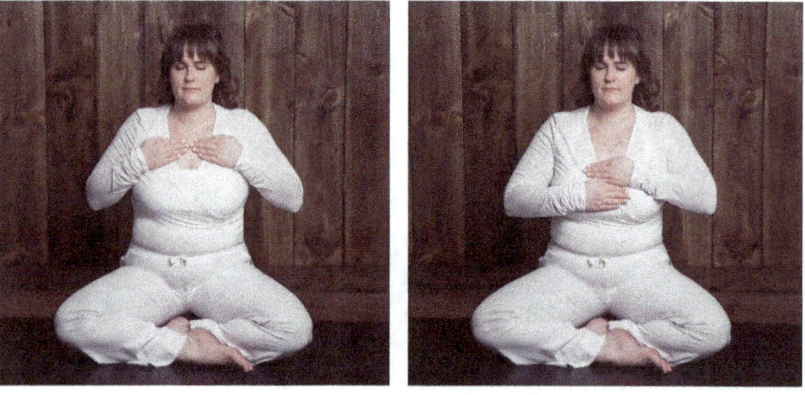

Pectorals, heart: place your hands on each pectoral, just below the collar bones. *Chakra: Heart.*

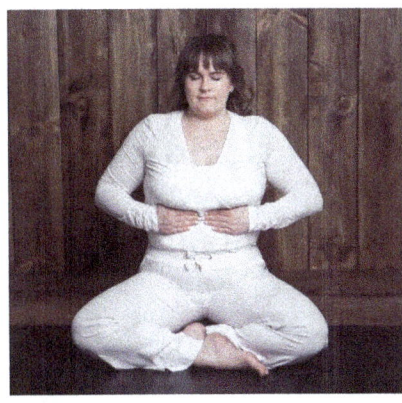 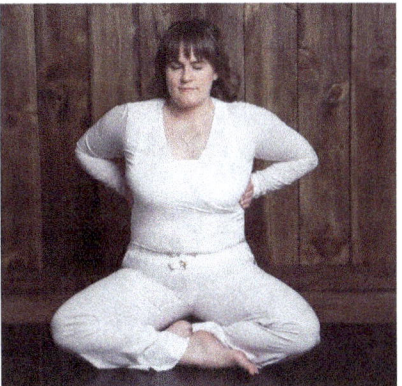

Ribs: place your hands on your ribs (just below the pectorals/breasts), then move your hands to the side like you are holding your rib cage (breathe into your hands). *Chakra: Heart.*

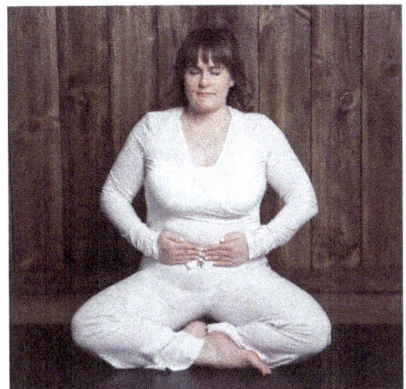 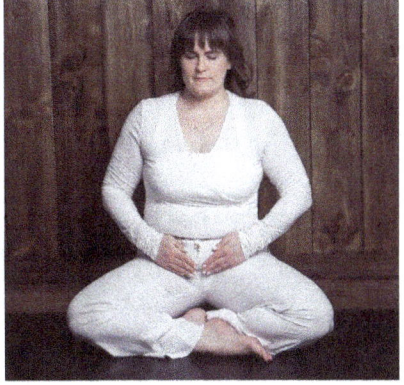

Low belly: place your hands on your lower abdomen, below the navel. Move your hands intuitively on the lower belly. *Chakra: Sacral.*

Abdomen: place one hand on abdomen (solar plexus, just below the ribs, centre from stomach) and one on your navel. Move your hands intuitively on the belly. *Chakra: Solar Plexus.*

BACK

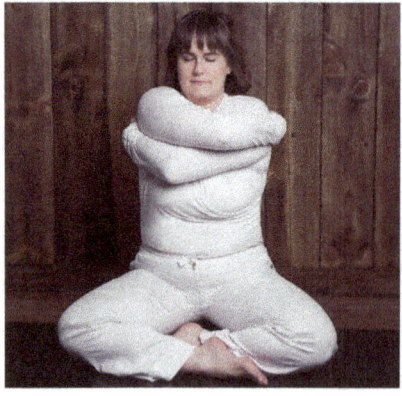 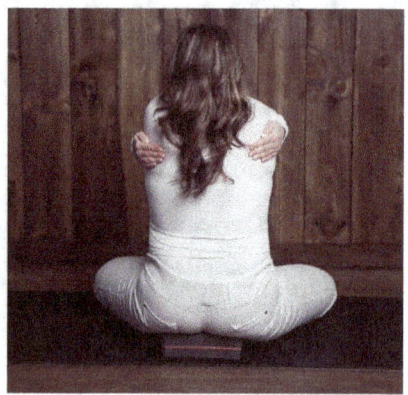

Scapulas: give yourself a hug, placing your hands on each shoulder blade. Switch sides. Offer yourself neck movements, play with the height of your elbows, and with the extension/folding/rolling/side bending of your spine, though if you are sitting still, your spine should be extending upward. *Chakras: Heart, and possibly Throat, Solar Plexus, Sacral.*

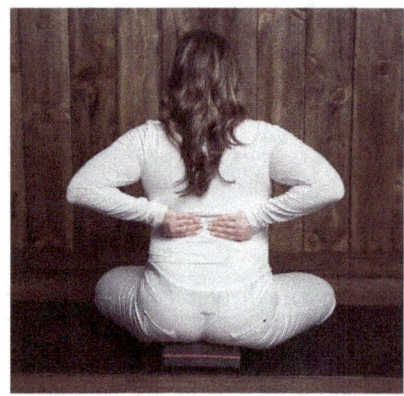 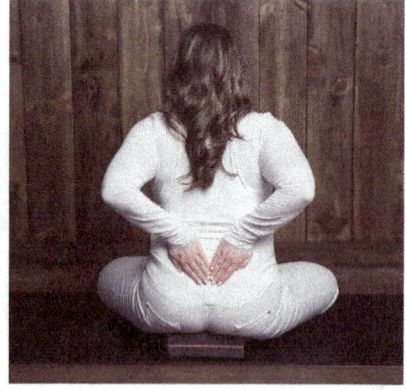

Mid-back: reach behind you and place your hands on your back ribs.

Low back and sacrum: place your hands on your low back, near your hips. Then move your hands to your sacrum (the bony part just before your glutes). *Chakra: Sacral.*

HIPS, LEGS, FEET

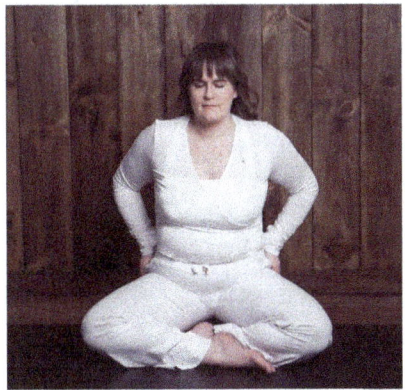 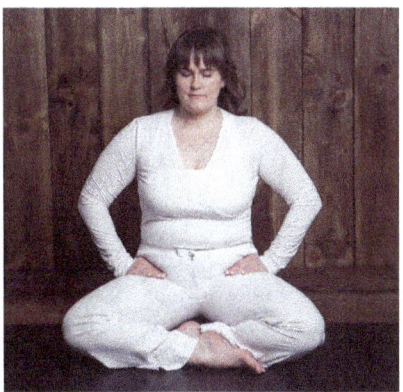

Hips: place your hands on the back, the side and the front of your hips, and move to the hip crease as well. *Chakras: Sacral, Root.*

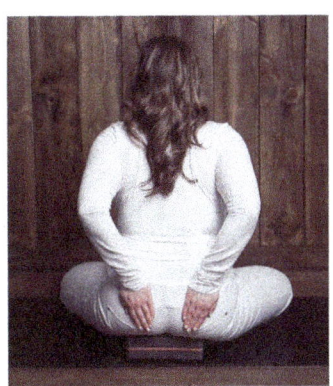

Glutes: place your hands on the top of the glutes muscles, and move intuitively; these are large muscles! *Chakra: Root.*

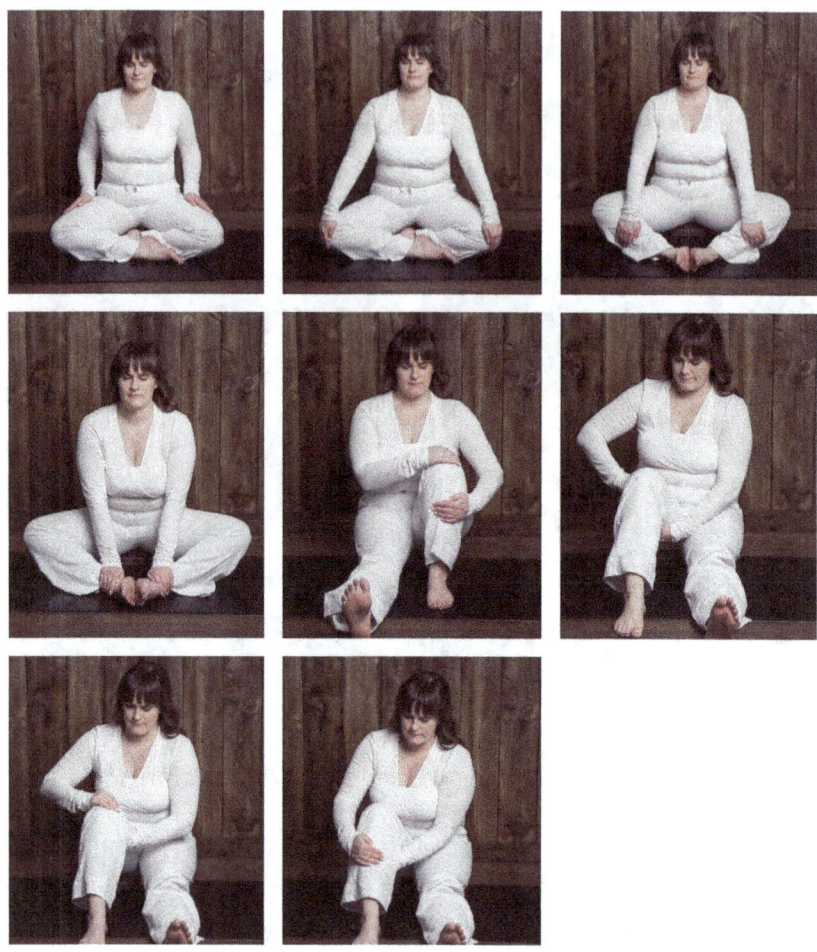

Legs: place your hands at different spots all around your thighs. Then move to your knees (front, side and back), shins and calves, and lastly, ankles and feet. *Chakra: Root.*

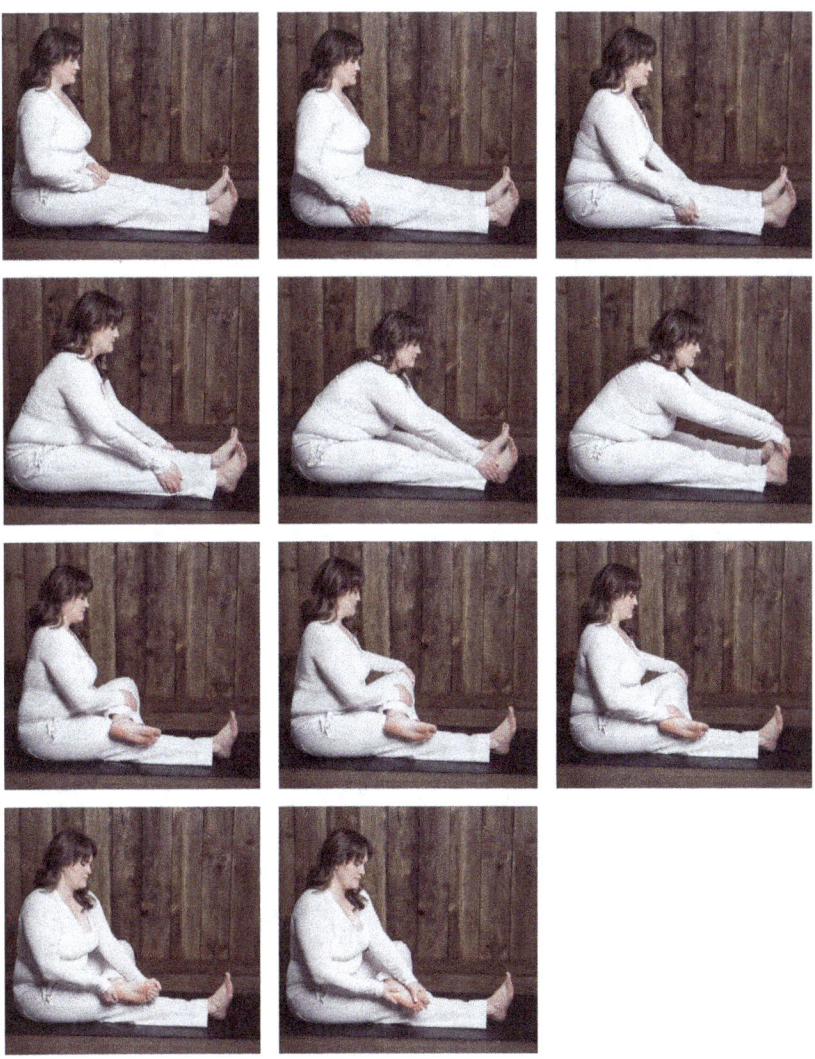

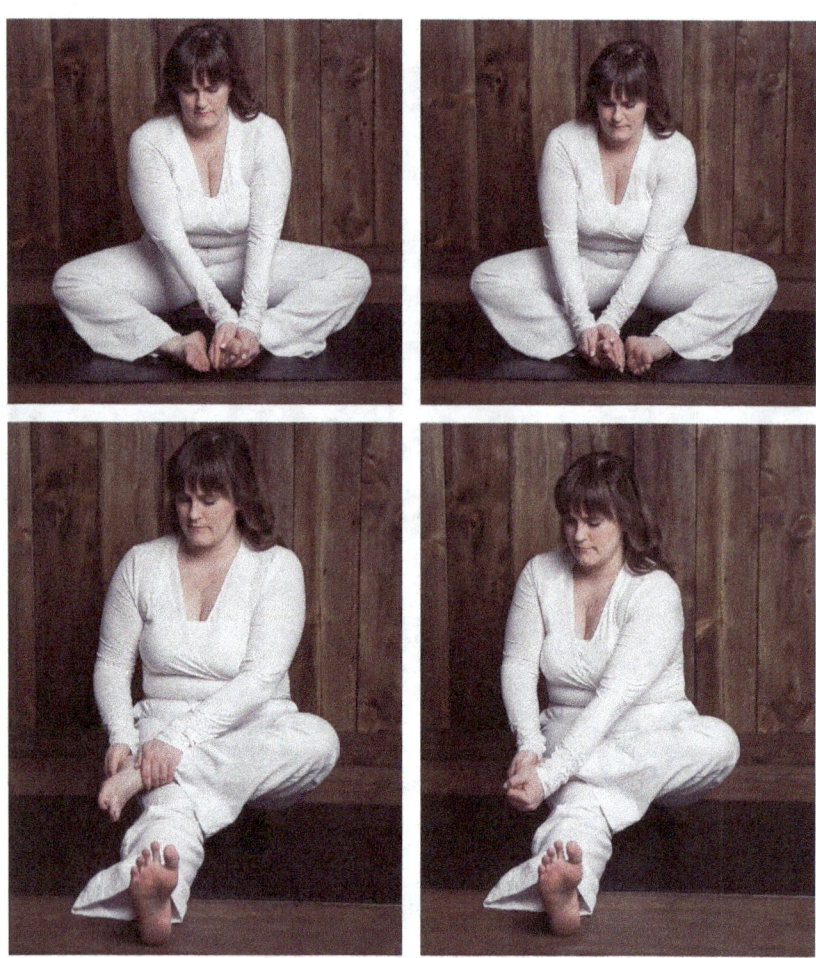

Feet: You can place hands intuitively, but I like to place one hand on the heel and the other on the toes, and one hand over, one hand under the arch. *Chakra: Root.*

MOVEMENT AND ASANAS

Every Reiki yoga class includes movement, whether traditional asanas or simple stretches (or both). This is the part of practice where yoga shines; it provides the physical outlet the body craves, and this applies in both gentler and more active practices.

I tend to punctuate my Reiki self-treatment with moving transitions and pepper hand positions into my asanas, making the experience a true hybrid of both methods.

ADAPTING THE POSES FOR REIKI TREATMENT

Any yoga posture can be supported by Reiki self-treatment! The only physical limitation is whether your own hands can reach the area you wish to touch in order to direct the Reiki energy. That being said, the base of your pose must be stable and your alignment must be safe. Beyond what our hands can reach, we can use the power of visualization, mindful breath and feeling, as well as sound to direct the energy where needed.

I know the analytically minded will question how sound-based energy can possibly carry light-based energy (as reiki is taught) because "sound and light are not the same nature". The answer lies in transmutation; everything is energy, therefore, "light" reiki which is taught as visual and touch, can change shape and travel as breath and sound. This is easier to understand when we remember that yoga calls breathwork "pranayama" (breath control or exercise) or more aptly, "the control of life energy". In my experience, visualization usually is the easiest way (and most commonly understood method) for beginners to send Reiki healing light to a body part, muscle, organ, or even a chakra. It is however important to note that energy is mutable, which means that other methods work too.

I personally use my inhale breath to "fuel the fire" of the healing light I'm channelling (whether it is Usui or Blue Star Reiki, or another form of light energy—more on that later when I discuss the light colours) and my out breath to expand the light and send it to the intended area. If I am channelling Reiki for my own self-treatment, I tend to use a few breaths to encourage the flow within my body (in breath is the masculine energy, out breath is the feminine energy, completing the flow cycle) and then use my inhale breath as the full body Reiki flow, and the out breath as the directive light to the intended area.

I then focus on the intended area, allowing my inhales to grow the light (i.e., make it brighter, more luminous) and my exhales to expand the light in and around the area (i.e., amplify and spread the light). For example, if I am treating my belly or my back, I will visualize the infinite flow of Reiki through my head down to the Earth (in breath), and looped back through my feet, up to the sky (out breath).

Then, I picture this figure-eight circuit flowing through my body on my inhale, and I see the light then travelling to my belly or back (either directly in my mind, or from my hands, in my mind—both are effective).

And lastly, I focus my inhales on seeing a brighter Reiki white light at the centre of my belly or back, and my exhales serve to expand the glow from the core to every cell and outward to surround my belly or back, until I feel it is iridescent.

In advanced Reiki yoga practice, we can use this technique to channel the Reiki first, then intentionally transfer it to someone (with respect for their free will, and an alternate redirection of the Reiki energy, if not accepted by the intended recipient), similarly to the Meditation to Transfer Healing Energy, in the kundalini yoga tradition (more on that in the Energy Healing Meditations section).

We can also use sound to send healing, as vibrations resonate with our cells (and our chakras). We can use traditional Reiki symbols sounded out (Cho Ku Rei, Sei Hei Ki, Hon Sha Ze Sho Nen) or any of the traditional hatha or kundalini yoga mantras, depending on our intention. I've recorded how I sound out the Usui symbols on my YouTube channel for inspiration.

BREATH AND MEDITATION

Breath is life. Yoga believes breath to be the drawing of both air *and* prana into the body. I use breath consciously throughout any yoga practice, regardless of style, but I also use it to encourage the flow of Reiki, and "feed the (inner) fire" so to speak.

It also helps my students follow the path of Reiki in their body. I guide practitioners to envision the Reiki flowing down through their body toward the Earth (yang or masculine energy) on the inhale, loop in the Earth, and drawing up through their body toward the Sky on the exhale (yin or female energy).

As for the path of Reiki, it moves into a figure-eight pattern; it enters the Crown (i.e., the top of the skull) flows down the front body, down the back of the legs and the feet, then from the Earth up the front of the feet and legs, up the back and spine, and out the Crown toward the Sky.

Practitioners also visualize, focus and feel, the up-turn of the Reiki flow simultaneously move down each arm and out their hands to "channel" and target areas of the (physical and/or energy) body during the (self-) treatment.

Following the breath is a meditation in and of itself. That said, I also occasionally add mantras (mentally or spoken), chants, breathing techniques (i.e., pranayama) and guided meditations to the Reiki activation and closing breaths. This is a type of practice that lends itself beautifully to meditation, both for beginners and more advanced yogi(ni)s and Reiki practitioners.

PRANAYAMA – BREATH EXERCISES

Of course, our breath is ever present, though much is gained from returning our attention to it, and even exploring *pranayama*, or "breath exercises." Breath is present in both the visualization and the sounding of energy. It can also be its own tool through the use of specific breaths. For instance, the famous "breath of fire" (agni pran) is absolutely a solar plexus / abdominal directed breath, whereas alternate nostril breath (nadi shodhana) is more of a third eye chakra / sinus / brain hemispheres balancing breath. If pranayama, or the "control of life force," speaks to you, I encourage you to explore this rich world of millenia-old wisdom, and this tool that already exists within you.

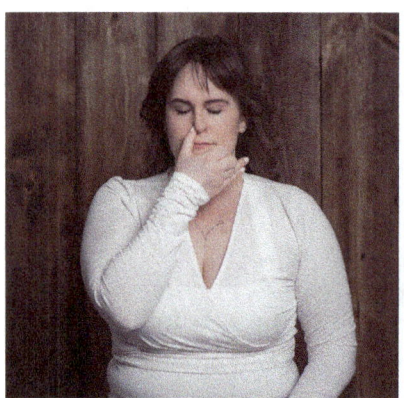 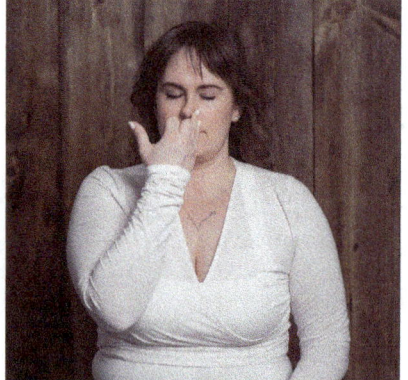

Nadi Shodhana—Alternate Nostril Breath

From a chakra yoga perspective, postures in and of themselves direct the energy; hence, the choice of a pose will help the energy flow and stimulate a particular (or a few) chakras. For example, postures that target the hips, low belly, and back tend to activate the second, sacral chakra, the centre of movement, creativity, sensuality, feminine energy, receptivity, and adaptability. Represented by water, it is the ultimate "going with the flow" chakra. When we practise poses that engage our legs, like lunges, balancing on one leg, squats like Goddess (Utkata Konasana), or poses that are low to the ground and deeply rooted, naturally stimulate the first or "root" chakra. Our base chakra deals with our physicality, our immediate needs, our safety, our relationship with money and family patterns.

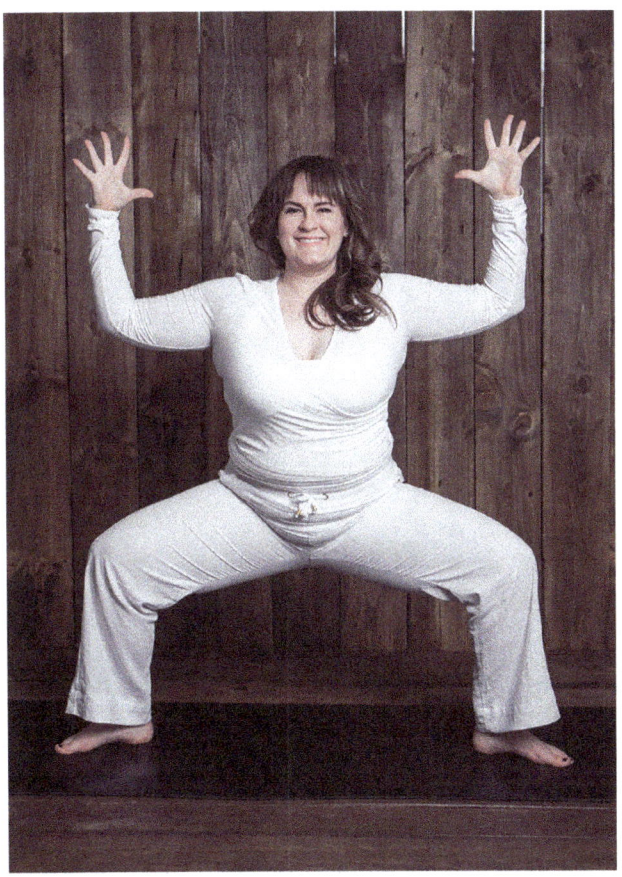

The first chakra is represented by matter and is the ultimate "stability" chakra. These are just a few examples of how to use poses to direct your energy. This is an intuitive process; trust your body's wisdom and trust yourself.

Chakra Pranayama to Balance Energy

CHAKRA ACTIVATED	ELEMENT	CHAKRA PRANAYAMA
Root	Matter/Earth	Sitting cross-legged. Inhale knees and arms up, exhale pull fists and knees down and sound out "HA!"
Sacral	Water	Sitting cross-legged. Inhale rock the pelvis forward, exhale rock it back.
Solar Plexus	Fire	Sitting cross-legged, hands resting on your knees. Inhale draw a circle forward with your torso, exhale draw it back to complete the circle. Do both directions.
Heart	Air	Sitting cross-legged, fingertips atop shoulders. Inhale twist your torso to the right, exhale twist left (a gentle whip movement). Do both directions.
Throat	Sound	Sitting cross-legged, hands interlaced under the jaw, elbows out. Inhale elbows up, pressing the jaw onto your hands gently. Exhale lever your chin up as your bring your forearms together, opening your throat. Sound out "aaah."
Third Eye	Light	Sitting, closed fingertips resting on your third eye (point between your eyebrows, at the base of your forehead), eyes closed. Inhale open your arms and eyes as if you were opening a curtain and look up. Exhale bring your head back to neutral, close your eyes, close the curtains by bringing your fingertips back onto your brow point.
Crown	Silence/Ether/Divine	Sitting, hands pressed together in prayer (anjali mudra). Inhale your joint hands up along the centre of your body and overhead, exhale open your hands up and arms over and around your sides, as through drawing a fountain of energy from your centre and enveloping you.

Inspired by Anodea Judith's Chakra Yoga exercises

SOUND: FROM YOGA TO REIKI, CHANTING AND MUSIC

The general definition of "sound" is that it is comprised of vibrations that travel through space (air or other medium) and can be heard when they reach a being's ears, or recorded by an audio device. Technically, a vibration is unique, and a frequency is the speed at which the vibration moves. What we recognize as harmonious sounds are higher frequency vibrations than unpleasant, choppy, off-key notes, for example.

Admittedly, this is a basic understanding of sound, but it has had an important role in yogic culture in both the Hatha and Kundalini traditions (e.g., bhakti yoga is all about devotion, universal love and praising through music).

Religions the world over have turned to song to pray and celebrate, both spiritually and emotionally healing practices (that isn't counting the science of recorded miracles, which is another topic altogether).

Indigenous Wisdom Keepers will tell you that singing and dancing are gateways to well-being and happiness; your body, its memory and its energetic layers, have a critical role in healing afterall! Befriending our bodies through movement and song is a simple principle with untapped potential.

In recent years, even western science has begun pouring over the idea that sound and music have a significant impact of physical and mental health. It's no wonder then that sound healing has been on the rise in our 'noisy' world, despite it being around in ancient cultures for millenia.

THE HEALING POTENTIAL OF SOUND: VIBRATION AND VOICE

The vibrations sound create, whether experienced from the outside in, or the inside out, have the potential to transform not only our energy fields (e.g., our moods, our energy levels, etc.) but also our cells and DNA.

Studies in the 1920s that recently resurfaced involving Rife machines demonstrated that certain frequencies could cure cancer by eradicating cancer cells while not killing healthy ones. A recent study showed that the regular practice of yoga and meditation could alleviate depression by helping to reverse the DNA damage that caused the mental illness. Now imagine combining the two? Powerful.

Singing a few minutes daily has been found to reduce cortisol levels (the stress hormone), exercises your lungs, abdominal and intercostal muscles and diaphragm, improves circulation, releases endorphins (the happy hormones). As we know, breath is life force, so if singing can improve the quality of your breathing it can improve your overall health.

Professor Graham Welch, Director of Educational Research at the University of Surrey, in Roehampton, UK said:

> Singing makes us breathe more deeply than many forms of strenuous exercise, so we take in more oxygen, improve aerobic capacity and experience a release of muscle tension as well.

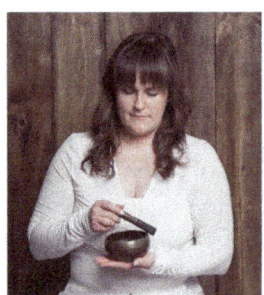 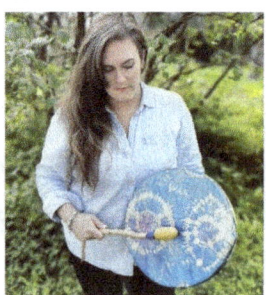 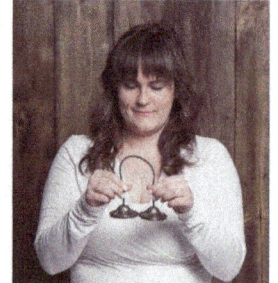

SOUND IN YOGA

Traditionally, both hatha and kundalini yoga teachings incorporate sound as a prana (life energy) driving modality. Yogis chant mantras, from simple bijas (or seed sounds) to phrases, in simple meditation or as part of pranayama (a breath exercise). Typically, in hatha, yogis will tone "Om" to open and close practice, which is the universal vibration, sound of creation and purifying the ego. There are several yogic prayers (affirmations) and kirtan chants (live group devotional music) in sanskrit as well.

In kundalini, yogis will often meditate—and do breathwork—to the mantra "sat nam" (translated to "my true essence"), and open their meditations with "ong namo guru dev namo" (translated to "I bow to the teacher within," calling upon the highest consciousness to guide the practice). In the western practice of kundalini, the song *Long Time Sun* has been a popularized devotion song. Here are the words:

> May the long time sun, shine upon you
> All love, surround you
> And may the pure light within you,
> Guide your way on, guide your way on,
> Sat nam, sat nam, sat nam.

Sound is a powerful tool that lives within us; our bodies can literally make music! I frequently tell my clients that chanting shakes off the energetic dust from the inside out, rippling through our energy field (aura). This is especially fascinating when you break down the process of chanting; you breathe in more air to project a sound, which means you take in more energy (chi/prana), and singing requires more air than speaking. Better quality breathing increased in the day-to-day means a better potential for healing (homeostasis). Ergo, singing helps heal you not only because it makes you happy, but because it forces you to breathe deeply.

BIJA MANTRAS
The sound behind each chakra

BIJA MANTRAS, OR "SEED SOUND" mantras, which are unique one-syllable sounds associated with our energy centres, are effective for chakra health and balancing (see the sound table included here for more details). Mantras can be expressed silently, in one's mind, but their power increases significantly when they are spoken, chanted, and even shared through group practice. I have fond memories of my hatha teacher training's kirtans (community devotion songs, in the bhakti branch of yoga) and our farewell "om canon." Our voices are a gift, a medicine within, and together, we are unspeakably, but audibly, powerful.

Chakras and Seed Sounds

CHAKRA	BIJA MANTRA (Seed sounds)
Root (Muladhara)	LAM
Sacral (Svadhisthana)	VAM
Solar Plexus (Manipura)	RAM
Heart (Anahata)	YAM
Throat (Vishuddha)	HAM
Third Eye (Ajna)	OM
Crown (Sahasrara)	OM, MAH

SOUND IN REIKI

AS FAR AS I have learned, Reiki isn't as closely linked to sound in its Usui lineage. This might be because Reiki is taught primarily as a light-based energy, not as a sound-based energy. But as mentioned earlier in this manual, sound is just another form energy can take, thus it can be used to encourage the flow of Reiki, and I dare say, all modalities of healing energy.

In Reiki treatments however, practitioners will often use tingshas (Tibetan bells on a string), Tibetan or crystal bowls to tone the beginning and end of a treatment. Sometimes, they use crystal bowls for each chakra tone, and may use their preferred sound tool over a troubled area, offering a sort of sound massage. Indigenous shamanic traditions use drums, rattles, chimes, clapping and song to restore energetic balance. Sound is a skillful complement to Light, in terms of energy healing. This is especially interesting if one considers that from an energetic perspective, all energy can be transmuted and take on many forms.

That being said, the beauty and effectiveness of Reiki lies in its simplicity. As a simple method that can be practised at any level, but mastered with dedicated practice over time, it lends itself well to interdisciplinary approaches and other energy work and healing paths. It's quite common to see Reiki Masters who are also intuitive channelers and healers, or even shamanic practitioners. Case in point, my first Reiki teacher, Deborah Fish, is a psychotherapist.

Silence is also a powerful practice that leaves space for observation and introspection. Finding a balance between using sound and silence intentionally in our practice is artful and rewarding. Through experimenting with sound and silence, we learn to overcome fears around producing sound (i.e., expressing ourselves fearlessly and truthfully), and similarly, about facing ourselves without distraction (i.e., who are we when we tune out the noise?).

REIKI SYMBOLS AS MANTRAS

Usui Reiki has a few symbols, which are bestowed upon its practitioners during their attunements (or "initiation ceremonies"). These symbols have names, and as my experience and my humble indigenous learnings have taught me, words hold power. I personally lead my Reiki yoga students (as well as my Reiki clients) in sounding out these symbols as a mantra, when I sense that the symbol could be beneficial to them.

In the Reiki tradition, practitioners would simply draw the symbol in the air, over a client (or onto, with their permission). Toning a symbol is another way of activating it, and I believe it is a way of embodying its power. The three Usui symbols I sound out with my students are Sei Hei Ki, Cho Ku Rei, and Hon Sha Ze Sho Nen. Generally, these are for emotional, physical, and distance/time (or "generational") healing. These symbols, which you can easily look up online, or learn about in *Essential Reiki* by Diane Stein or in the *Reiki Manual* by Penelope Quest, are simple yet powerful symbols that act on several levels, echoing through our four energy bodies (body, emotions, mental, spiritual). Please study them, treat them with respect and you will not use them "incorrectly." Since there is no rulebook on the tone of these symbols, I do so intuitively, while respecting the correct pronunciation of course!

Usui Reiki Symbols As Mantras

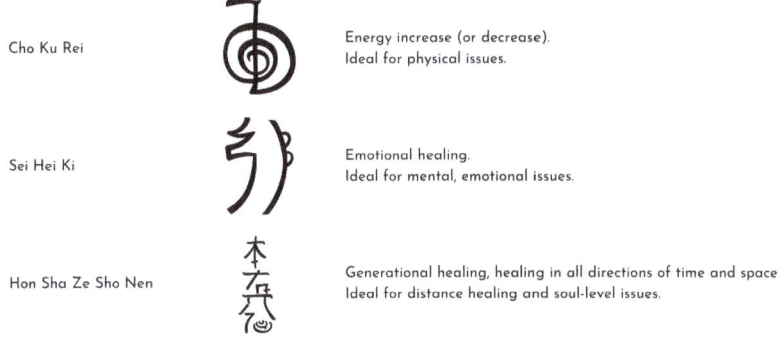

Cho Ku Rei — Energy increase (or decrease). Ideal for physical issues.

Sei Hei Ki — Emotional healing. Ideal for mental, emotional issues.

Hon Sha Ze Sho Nen — Generational healing, healing in all directions of time and space. Ideal for distance healing and soul-level issues.

MUSIC

As discussed so far, sound is a powerful tool; rhythm, melody, notes and tone, chanting words (mantras), and playing an instrument all carry fascinating medicine. Yet, the best tools are always the most personal; the ones that resonate with us, the ones we feel called to use and of course, our own natural abilities and skills as these make for a customized, embodied experience.

In other words, silence, our voice, our bodies, and perhaps instruments to which we are particularly drawn, are often the best choices for us as Reiki yoga practitioners, and perhaps as sound healers. Our bodies hold some of the most potent sound medicine, so to speak. I would compare live music and recorded music to fresh, homemade food, and pre-packaged or restaurant meals. You can have poor or great quality in either scenario, but the odds are the fresh food will have the greatest benefits and most nutrients, if not necessarily the gourmet appeal. Essentially, the first-hand (embodied) experience is unmatched for sound healing potential.

That said, if you feel called to use recorded music, do so mindfully, not just because silence is uncomfortable. One could argue that for that very reason, befriending silence would become the practice.

When you do play recorded music, do so intentionally. There are wonderful conscious musicians and sound healers out there who produce beautiful music and soundscapes. I encourage you to find artists you admire (whether on YouTube, recommended by friends or teachers you respect, or by simply consulting a local New Age bookshop for a few old-school CD suggestions and a sample listen in store or online). Find artists with whom you align and support their work by purchasing the tracks you love. I personally enjoy instrumental pieces from wellness and spirituality companies like Gaiam, New Age artists like Loreena McKennitt, and yoga music from artists such as Deva Premal, Mirabai Ceiba, and Edo & Jo. Spa and massage therapy music or nature sounds would also be lovely options.

INTEGRATION AND GRATITUDE

Savasana is the traditional integration pose for all yoga classes. It is therefore a great time to reconnect to the Reiki energy and take a moment to send our gratitude for its support of our bodies and practice. It's important to "unplug" from the flow, as a means of respect, knowing that whenever we need it, we can mindfully connect. It's also the time to release our Reiki guides from the sacred space created, and send them our thanks as well. We assess how we're feeling and we let go in trust. We bring our awareness back and collect ourselves, to then close practice. I recommend closing with a chant, such as Om Shanti, Shanti, Shanti, Om (or Om Reiki, Om Shanti, Om).

PART 2 HIGHLIGHTS

THE COMPONENTS of a Reiki yoga practice:

- Creating sacred space
- Grounding and Intention
- Reiki activation (meditation)
- Body scanning
- Self-treatment and hand positions
- Movement and postures
- Mindful breath and meditation
- Hand position assists (personal or as teacher-facilitator)
- Sound (mantras, song, instruments, music, soundscape, silence)
- Integration and gratitude

CONSIDERATIONS FOR YOUR REIKI YOGA PRACTICE

MINDFULNESS AND VIPASSANA

AS WITH MANY WELLNESS TRADITIONS, the benefits of Reiki yoga (and meditation) are reaped over time, expanded through experience and are ultimately an embodied practice. Reiki yoga is a newer expression of two healing arts and holistic approaches to being human, to being light living in a body. But at its core, Reiki yoga is an exercise in mindfulness as it solicits all physical senses and fosters intuition, while providing physical, mental, emotional, and spiritual benefits.

Mindfulness is the practice of being present and aware of one's own thoughts, feelings, behaviours, and reactions. It's also about understanding the relationships between our experiences and impermanent states of being, for instance, noticing what causes our moods to change.

In the yogic tradition, mindfulness is called "vipassana," which translates in English to "clear seeing," refers to the insight into the true nature of reality. Vipassana is a meditation involving concentration on the body or its sensations, as well as passing thoughts and feelings, and on another level, it is observing the insights these provide.

CHAKRAS

You can also approach your Reiki yoga practice from the perspective of chakras. Since Reiki is energy work, and chakras are energy centres, it makes sense to proceed from an energetic perspective.

In other words, where is energy (not) flowing? What areas of your life need more attention? Then build your Reiki yoga practice around the chakras that appear to be deficient (or excessive).

Chakras in the Body

Chakra	Root	Sacral	Solar Plexus	Heart	Throat	Third Eye	Crown
Sanskrit Name	Muladhara	Svadhisthana	Manipura	Anahata	Vishuddha	Ajna	Sahasrara
Element	Matter	Water	Fire	Air	Sound	Light	Thought
Function	Survival, grounding	Desire, pleasure, sexuality, reproduction	Will, power, assertiveness	Love	Communication, creativity	Seeing, intuition	Understanding
Location	Base of the spine, perineum	Lower abdomen, womb, genitals	Navel to solar plexus	Heart	Throat	Eyebrow point, at the centre of the forehead	Top of the head
Body part	Legs, feet, bones, large intestine, teeth	Womb, genitals, kidney, bladder, circulatory system	Digestive system, muscles	Heart, lungs, pericardium, arms, hands	Neck, shoulders, ears, mouth	Eyes	Cerebral cortex, central nervous system
Glands	Adrenals	Ovaries, testes	Pancreas, adrenals	Thymus	Thyroid, parathyroid	Pineal	Pituitary
Sense	Smell	Taste	Sight	Touch	Hearing		

I recommend reading Anodea Judith's *Wheels of Life* to further learning on chakras, and her *Chakra Yoga* to learn more about the connection between yoga practice and chakra health. She explains how chakra imbalances manifest as illness, disorder and disease, and relates examples for each chakra. You can then explore further how Reiki and chakra yoga can be combined.

For the purposes of this manual, I have limited my examples of the chakras to the traditional seven, but once you begin mastering energy, you will inevitably discover there are thousands of small chakra points, and there are twelve major chakras, which authors such as Diana Cooper discusses in *The Twelve Chakras*, or Laurelle Shanti Gaia in her book, *Karuna Reiki®*.

LIGHT AND COLOURS

Traditional Usui Reiki is presented as a pure and infinite white light. Healing white light is also frequently referenced in kundalini yoga. Blue Star celestial Reiki is described as a galactic blue energy, meant for deep generational, shamanic healing, thus enabling travel through dimensions. In Karuna Reiki®, shades of pink represent the healing energy of unconditional love and compassion, inspired by Kuan Yin.

ANGEL RAYS

In the New Age and in modern energy work, practitioners talk about angel rays. These are said to be the energies of the archangels/archeia (the female counterparts to the recognized archangels) and their respective overseen areas of this life and beyond.

For example, the yellow ray is associated with Archangel Gabriel, while the green ray is associated with Archangel Raphael. Each ray has its children, and its dedicated practitioners (or "lightworkers," "energy healers," etc.). In other words, each soul journeying on Earth is watched over by an archangel/archeia "team," which we identify as a ray of colourful light energy. The people born to Archangel Raphael's ray of emerald light tend to be natural healers who feel drawn to help people around them, whether personally, professionally, or both. Archangel Michael's "team" watches over truth seekers and tellers with a strong sense of justice; these are often the people who lead peaceful protests and campaign for causes they stand behind. The blue ray of Archangel Michael may also include people in law enforcement, such as police officers and lawyers. If you feel drawn to learn about angel rays, you may want to read works by Radleigh Valentine, Kyle Gray, Diana Cooper or Claire Stone, as they've written extensively on angels.

Archangels and Archeia

Archangel	Archeia	Ray
Michael	Faith	First (1st), Blue, Protection, Faith, Will of the Creator/God/Universe
Jophiel	Christine	Second (2nd), Yellow, Wisdom and Illumination
Chamuel	Charity	Third (3rd), Pink/Rose, Divine Love
Gabriel	Hope	Fourth (4th), White, Purity and the Ascension Flame
Raphael	Mother Mary	Fifth (5th), Green, Truth, Healing, Abundance
Uriel	Aurora	Sixth (6th), Red, Service and Peace
Zadkiel	Holy Amethyst	Seventh (7th), Violet, Freedom, Transmutation, Forgiveness

NB: This table serves as a sample list, and experts would have more extensive details on each of the above as well as unlisted archangels and archeia.

THE COLOURS OF MOTHER EARTH AND FATHER SKY

When I meditate on the Earth Mother, Gaia, I tune into her core heartbeat and feel warm, pink, lava flowing, maternal love. If I need her physical healing, an energy boost, or to feel her abundance, I tune into her lush greens, whereas when I need emotional cleansing I tune into her deep blues for profound work and soothing turquoise for a calming effect. To ground myself, I imagine rich browns, and often see my energetic roots burrowing into the earth. Mother Earth is the Mama I turn to when I need comfort, healing, or support.

When I meditate on Grandmother Moon, I tune into her age-old wisdom and perspective, and I feel a fresh silver light, sometimes a beam, others more of a sparkle, which is calm, patient awareness and wisdom. I feel acceptance and compassion from this matriarch. She's the grandmother who offers a slice of solicited advice with a cup of tea.

When I tune into Grandfather Sun, I feel a loving, warm, generous patriarch that shines golden light. To me, he is the proud, protective grandfather who offers patronage and practical gifts.

When I tune into Father Sky, I tune into indigo blue starry sky and I feel inspired, driven, confident, abundant, encouraged by an expansive fatherly love. I have a similar feeling to being up on my father's shoulders, seeing the world from new heights.

Those are my personal experiences, and there is some level of essence to different energies, but we may still experience them based on our own perspectives.

Psychologists led studies on the effect of colours, but that's just scratching the surface of colour therapy and energy. Light and colours have different vibrations and therefore act on specific levels of energy bodies, and types of wounds or issues that requiring healing.

Now that you know that chakras have colours, and there are angel rays, and different types of Reiki energies available, feel free to explore the meaning of colours and try to visualize them flowing into (and out of) your body, as you would traditional white light

Usui Reiki energy. This will give you a range of powerful positive energy to support your Reiki yoga practice, as well as your meditation practice. You can choose to actively learn about colour therapy, chakra associations, and/or angel rays. This will enable you to choose colours to work with, or even to start looking for colours within your body to "see" what needs attention, and potential healing.

You can also let yourself discover other colour energies intuitively as they come up in your own practice, for example, when you are scanning or laying hands on your body. This intuitive approach to colourful light energies means that you don't influence your intellectual understanding of a colour, and you let the feeling or impression teach you. Both of these approaches are valid, interesting and effective!

Healing Lights

Healing Light Colour	Associated Energies
White	Universal healer, Purity, Divine, Life force.
Gold/Silver	Divine Masculine (Sun/Sky/Air/Fire) / Divine Feminine (Earth/Moon/Water/earth element), Divine Healing.
Violet	Magic, Wisdom, Divine connection, Spirituality, Inspiration.
Indigo/Deep blue	Calm, Vision, Dreams, Water medicine, Unseen, the Ocean.
True blue, turquoise	Healthy communication, Truth, Justice, Water medicine, the Sky.
Green	Growth, Healing, Nature's medicine, Mother Earth.
Pink/Rose	Mother Earth, Femininity, Fertility, Nurturing, All forms of Love, Sisterhood.
Yellow	Confidence, the Sun, Joy, Empowerment.
Orange/Coral	Creativity, Flow, Pleasure/Playfulness, Receptivity.
Red	Vitality, Strength, Grounding, Abundance, Fire/Transformation.
Brown	Warm earthy connection, Grounding, Abundance.
Black	Mystery, Protection, Negativity transmutation, Wisdom.

*Your own associations and feelings about these colours, lights and energies will always be stronger than any convention. Trust yourself.

HYDRATION AND THE WATER CONNECTION

I often refer to Reiki as flowing like water, from the Infinite to the Earth's core, and back to the Infinite. In my meditations, I describe a waterfall of cascading (or trickling if that suits you better!) white light. Reiki is dynamic and "flows" like a stream or river, even though our eyes don't usually perceive movement in light.

Reiki energy circulates in a figure eight in our bodies, and as a "universal life force energy," it supports health, not unlike water! From my experience working with Reiki clients, hydration is key to assisting energy flow, but also, in alleviating any type of energy work's "detox symptoms," from headaches to digestive issues, fatigue and an emotional hangover.

I recommend in my hatha and yin classes to hydrate before and after practice (at least one hour prior, one hour after), because we work the tissues in a way that creates "space" for hydration. The body is effective and tends to use current patterns; without creating this space in the cells, we simply eliminate more of the extra water we drink without significantly improving our body's hydration.

Similarly, Reiki requires our bodies to be hydrated to gently assist in the flushing out of physical and energetic gunk (i.e., the stagnant energy that no longer serves a purpose in our well-being). This "flushing out process" is true for both a session of Reiki treatment as for a Reiki yoga practice.

MORNING WATER RITUAL INSPIRED BY GRANDFATHER DOMINIQUE RANKIN

YEARS AGO, I met Algonquin Wisdom Keeper Dominique Rankin, and he shared a teaching on water carrying energy. He suggested a morning water ritual based on the medicine wheel.

The Medicine Wheel

DIRECTION	MEDICINE WHEEL QUARTER	ELEMENT	ENERGIES INVITED
East	Yellow	Water	Life/Birth New Day, Rebirth, Renewal, Hope, Intention.
South	Red	Fire	Awareness, Self-respect, Integrity, Motivation, Respect for others.
West	Black	Earth	Acceptance, Forgiveness, Letting go, Understanding, Wisdom from experience.
North	White	Air	Healing, Inner Freedom, Peace, Love, Compassion, Perspective.

*These are general guidelines. Please feel free to explore what each quarter of the Medicine Wheel had to teach you.
**I have left out references to Spirit Animals in this table, as they vary greatly based on the Nation's culture and interpretation of the Medicine Wheel.

He taught me to pour a glass of fresh water as my first intentional action of the day. (I personally infuse it with Reiki as I meditate over it.) He instructed me to face East and drink to the new day, to rebirth and renewal. Turning to my right, facing South, I was to drink to self-awareness and self-respect. I would turn to my right to face West and drink to forgiveness and letting go. Lastly, I would turn to my right to face North and drink to peace and acceptance. Then I'd turn East again to start my day.

Here is my interpretation of this meditation. When you first get up, before starting your daily activities, pour a glass of fresh water, and mindfully hold it in both hands, visualizing Reiki white light infusing the water. Imagine yourself flowing with Reiki energy, standing in the centre of a medicine wheel, facing

East. Begin drinking water following the themes of each direction, inviting their positive energy into your body and into your energy field. Before turning to each direction, take a moment to visualize and feel each sip of water as increasing the flow of Reiki white light flowing within you.

Part Three

Sequences to Build Upon

REIKI YOGA SEQUENCES

THE SEQUENCES INCLUDED in this manual are not intended to be rigorously followed and never altered; as you journey and change, so does your practice evolve. Reiki yoga as a discipline, and your relationship to its practice will also transform over time and experience.

The sequences are thoughtfully crafted so that beginners can feel guided and build confidence, while allowing more advanced practitioners to use them for inspiration and further exploration.

SEQUENCE 1: GROUNDING
PRACTICE FOCUS BY AREA: LEGS & HIPS

THIS SEQUENCE ACTIVATES and balances the lower chakras. This includes the Earth, the root (or base, first) and sacral (second) chakras. The Earth chakra (located about one foot or 30 cm below your feet) connects us to Mother Earth, our primary instincts and our inner child or subconscious, and it acts as a portal to what shamanic traditions call the Lower World.

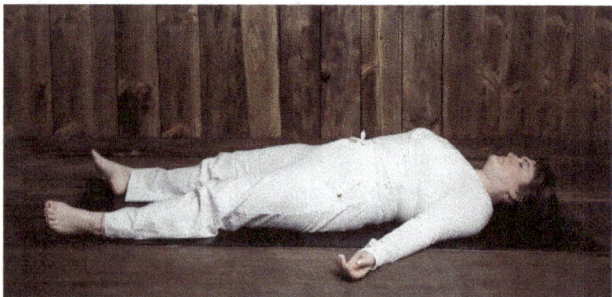

Savasana: lie flat on your back. If your low back is sensitive, support knees with a rolled blanket, bolster, or blocks, or simply bend the knees and place feet flat (ardha savasana)

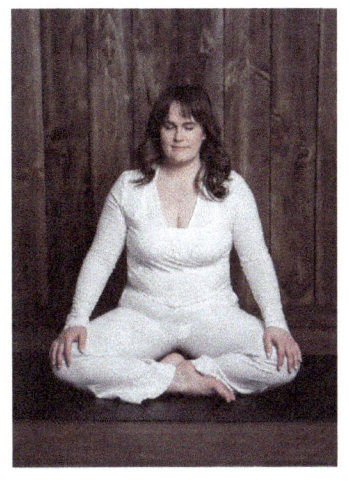

Reiki Meditation: Either lying down or seated, start deepening your breath. Eyes closed, visualize the infinite flow of Reiki white light. When ready, invite it into your body and encourage its figure-eight flow (down the front of your body, and the back of your legs, into the Earth, up the front of your legs and the back of your torso, out of your Crown toward the Sky). On your inhales, draw the light down; on your exhales, draw the light up, completing the pattern.

Body scan: Using cupped hands, hovering a few inches above/away from your body, start scanning your body (and energy field) from head to toe. Notice what comes up for you in terms of sensations, temperature, energy levels, mood, and emotions, and thoughts. It's an option to rub your palms together to call upon the Reiki energy and awaken your hands to better perceive and scan. You may wish to sit for this.

Upper body hand positions: Referring back to the upper body self-treatment hand positions, intuitively work your way from head to low back and belly and offer yourself a self-treatment. You may wish to sit for this portion to enable more comfortable reach for the hand positions.

Pelvis movements: Whether you are still lying down, or sitting comfortably, you can rock your pelvis gently, waking up the low back and belly. Inhale rock forward (arching your back), exhale rock back (eliminating the natural curve of the spine). Some say this stimulates the sacral chakra, our centre of feminine energy, creativity, and pleasure. Others say it awakens the kundalini energy, which is the coiled snake of female energy at the base of the spine.

This next portion works best lying down.

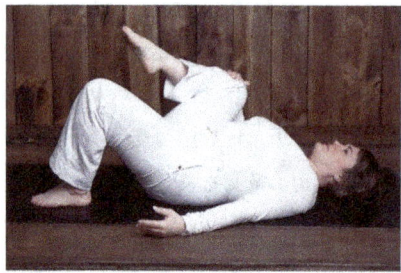 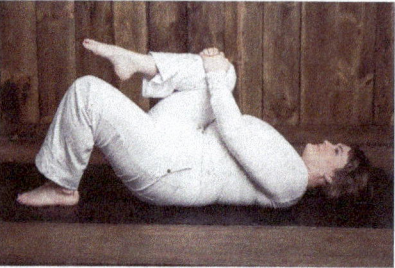

Hip and ankle circles: Take a moment to draw circles with your pelvis, hips and ankles.

- Hug your knees into your chest and rock side to side, and draw circles with your knees onto the sky.
- Resting one foot flat, hug one knee into the chest and with your hand(s) guide your knee to draw circles in the sky (in both directions) to warm up the hip.
- You may want to open the hip by sending the knee toward the outside (intending to the armpit) and keeping your hip on the ground, drawing the knee inward, stretching the outside of the thigh and glutes.
- While hugging your knee into your chest one last time, draw circles with your toes to warm up your ankle. Flex and point your foot as feels good.
- Do the other side.

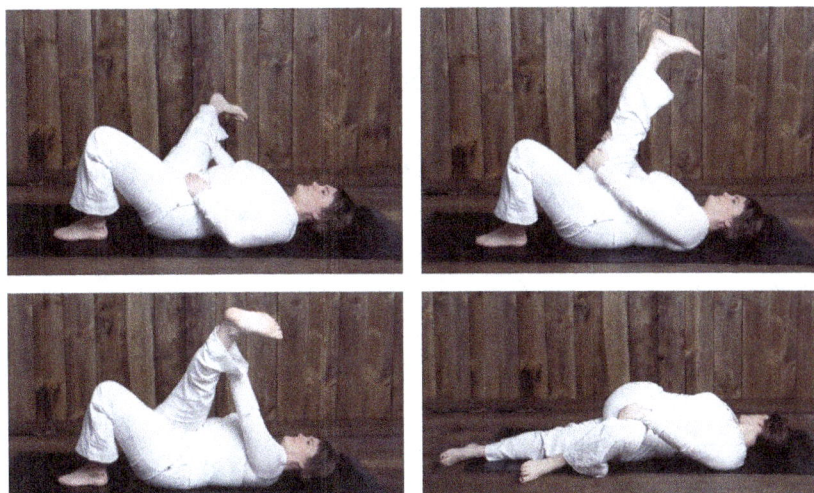

Leg stretches + supine twists: Returning to the first leg, you'll extend your leg to the sky, foot flexed (as if you're standing on the ceiling), with a gentle bend in your knee, fingers interlaced behind your thigh (or using a yoga strap around your foot. Tip: your shoulders and arms should be relaxed)

- Use your breath to guide the extent of your stretch (inhale to relax a little, exhale to draw the leg closer, deepening the stretch in the back of your leg and low back)
- Keeping both hips grounded on the mat, use your hands to guide the extended (or bent) leg into a hip opening (i.e., your leg goes toward the outside of your body). Bring the leg back to centre and bend the knee to your chest.

Use these two postures to intuitively offer yourself hand positions in the legs, knees, feet and low belly.

- Take your opposite hand and guide the leg across your body into a twist (your hip will inevitably lift off the ground). You may use a block or bolster to greet your twisting leg and support your lower back.

Take this opportunity to offer yourself hand positions of the hips, glutes, and thighs.

- Do the other side.

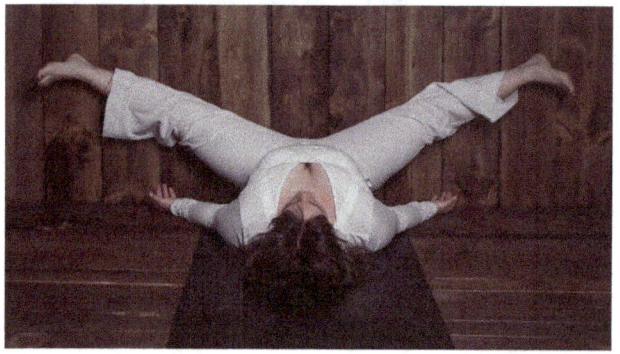

Open V Stretch: Using your hands to support your legs and guide the extent of the stretch that is comfortable for your mobility, allow both legs to open into a V shape. If this is too intense, you can keep the knees bent and hug your knees toward your armpits (e.g., like squatting, but on your back).

- If you feel comfortable holding this position for a few breaths, you can explore lower body and leg hand positions that feel right to you.
- Hug your knees into your chest, rock gently, and rest your feet flat on the mat.

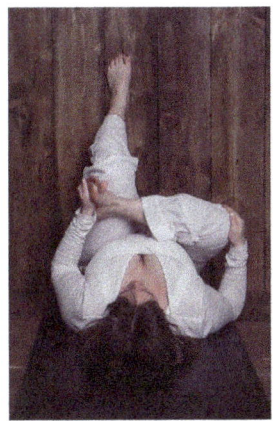 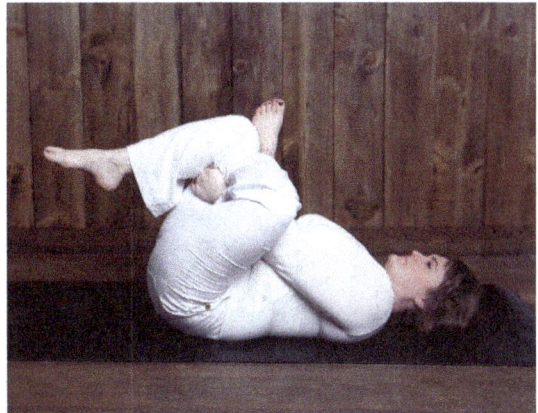

Figure 4 Stretch (Reclined Pigeon Variation): With one foot flat on the mat, extend the other leg skyward, gentle bend in the knee, foot flexed. From the hip, turn your heel slightly into your body (like you're trying to click your heels), bend the knee at a 90-degree angle and rest the flexed foot (important to protect the knee) onto the opposite thigh (i.e., the one whose foot is flat on the ground).

- You can rest your hands on the knee and foot of the leg in figure 4 and offer an organic self-treatment.
- You can choose to reach for the back of the opposite thigh to hug the legs in and deepen the stretch.

You always have the option to offer yourself intuitive hand positions.

- Do the other side.

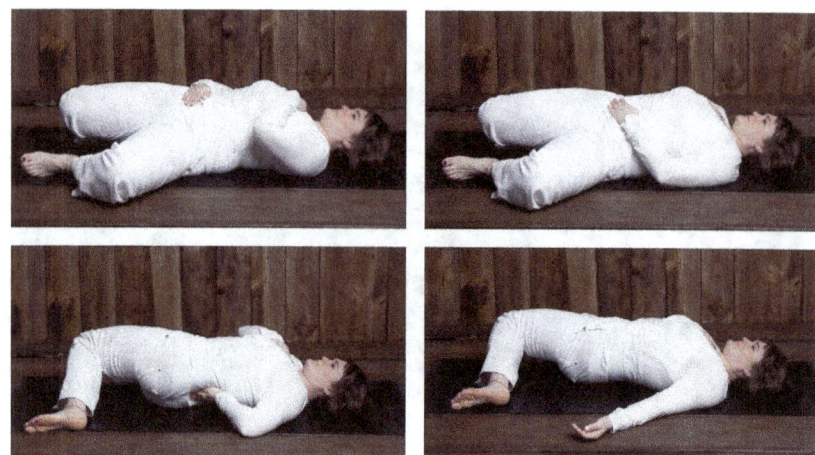

Windshield Wiper: Arms by your side (palms up), take a wide stance, allow your knees to fall from side to side. The wider your feet, the gentler this is on the lower back and the more you feel the movement in the hips.

- Coordinate your breath with your movement by inhaling the knees to centre, exhaling them to the side. Pausing as you need to, offering extra breaths.
- You can hug opposite elbows and allow your elbows to swing side to side, always opposing your knees, if that feels comfortable for you.
- When taking pauses, feel free to add any hand position that feels right. As windshield wiper is a twist, it is particularly suitable for torso self-treatment (front or back).

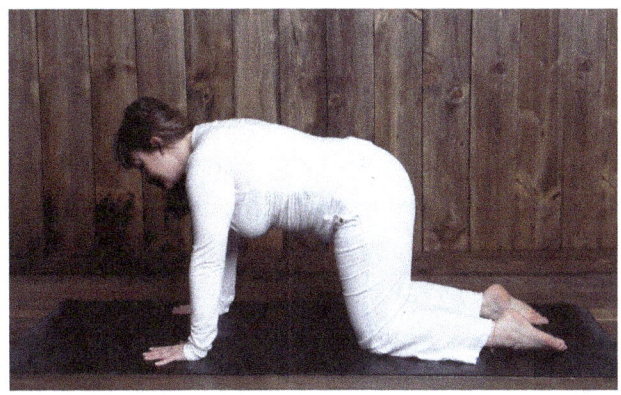

Rock Up To Table pose (Bharmanasana): Hug both knees into your chest, tuck your chin to your collarbone engaging your abdominals and start to rock back and forth along your spine, build momentum. If you feel comfortable, cross your ankles and when your sense the rocking is strong enough, come up to table pose, on all fours. Otherwise, slow the rocking, turn to your side, and use your hands to help yourself to a table.

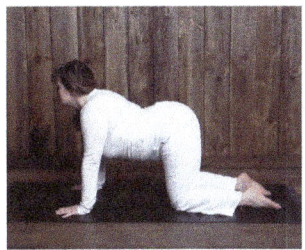 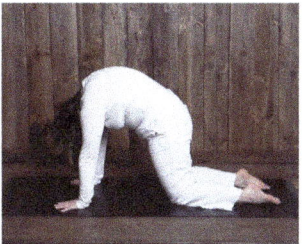

Cat-Cow (Marjaiasana and Bitilasana): Continue your spinal warm-up by inhaling the belly down, hugging the shoulder blades back, looking forward (not cranking the neck unnecessarily), tilting the pelvis forward to gently arch your back. Exhale, tuck in your navel to your spine, tilt your pelvis back sending your tailbone to the ground, round out your back and shoulders, and allow your head to drop. Follow this breath and movement for a few breaths, or as long as you need.

- *If you are pregnant, in postpartum recovery, or have had abdominal surgery, you may want to pay special attention to abdominal sensations and keep this movement small and gentle.*

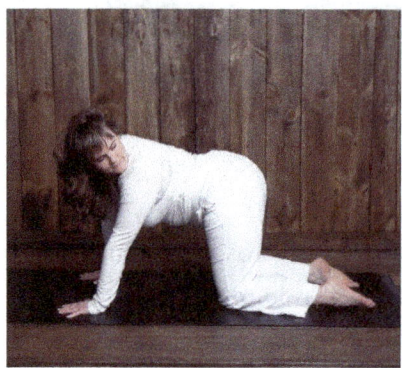 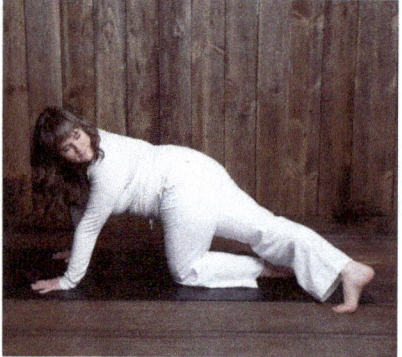

Dog Looking At Its Tail: on all fours in table pose, inhale with neutral spine. Exhale as you try to look behind you "at your tail," making this a gentle lateral stretch. Inhale back to neutral spine, and exhale to stretch the other side.

- Extend your leg back, toes curled under, pull the heel back on the exhale to stretch your calf.
- Cross your extended leg's foot over to your other side and try to look at your foot, into another lateral stretch.
- Do the other side.

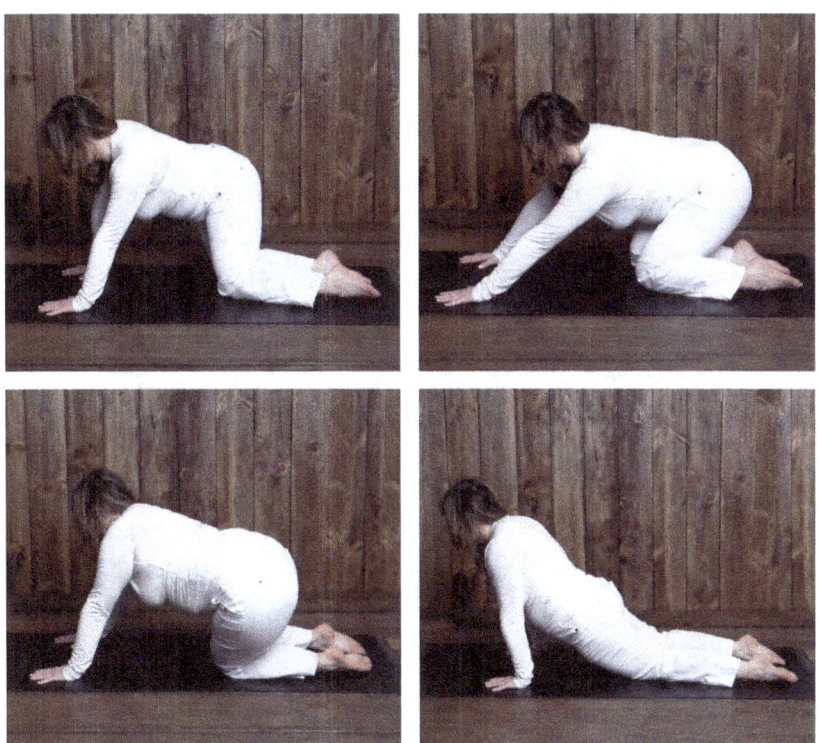

Hip circles: from table pose, sway your hips from side to side, then create a big "U" shape with your hips, into large hip circles. Do both sides.

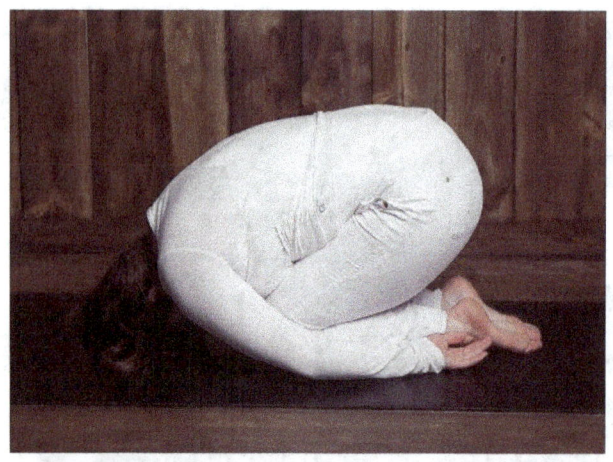

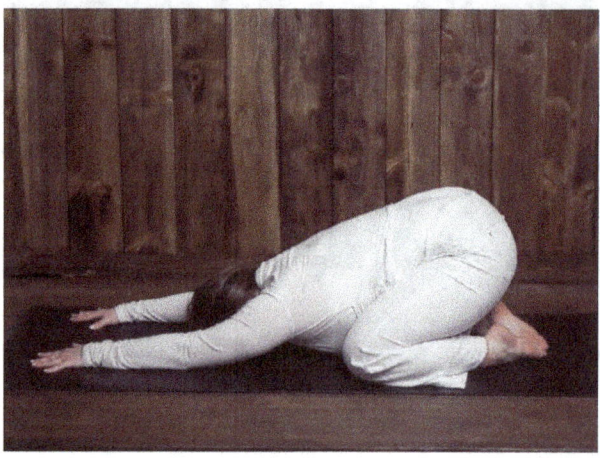

Child's pose, arms by your side. For a restorative option, add blocks under the front of the shoulders for support. For a hip opening effect, you can take this pose with wider knees.

CHILD'S POSE (BALASANA): from table pose, pull your hips back toward your heels and rest forward into child pose.

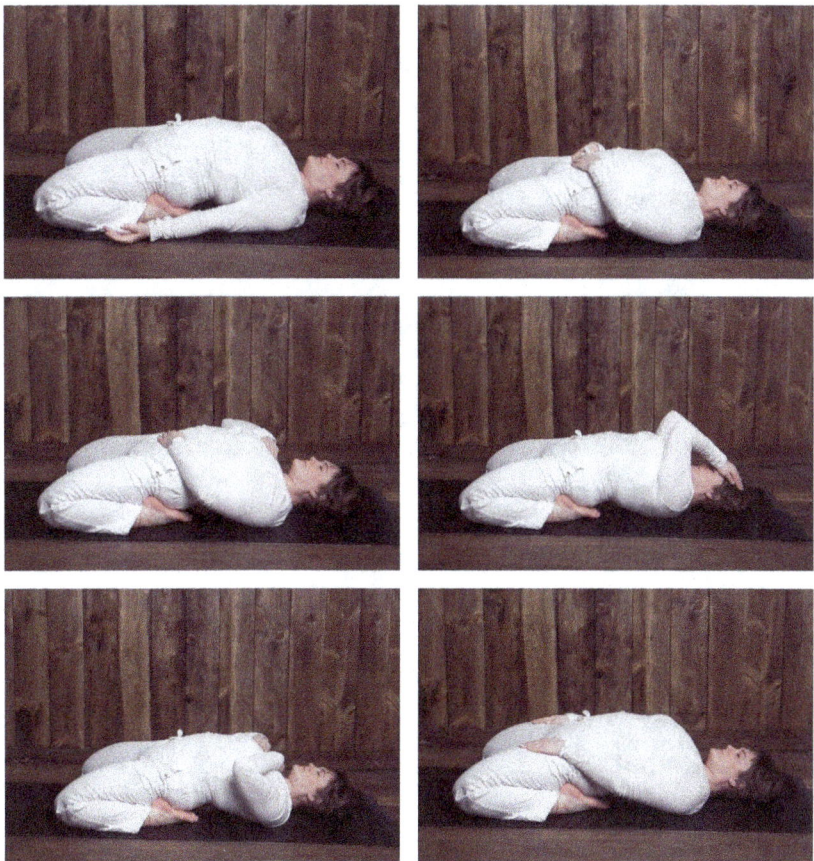

- For more advanced yogi(ni)s, who wish to take **Reclined Hero Pose (Supta Virasana)**, stay seated on your heels, allowing the heels to be at the outer edge of your thighs to allow space for your glutes. I recommend taking a bit wider with the knees to protect the lower back. Lean back onto hands, forearms onto blocks or the ground, or fully reclined, if this feels good for you. Take a few breaths here.
- Offer yourself a hand position intuitively. Use your arms to help yourself out of the pose.

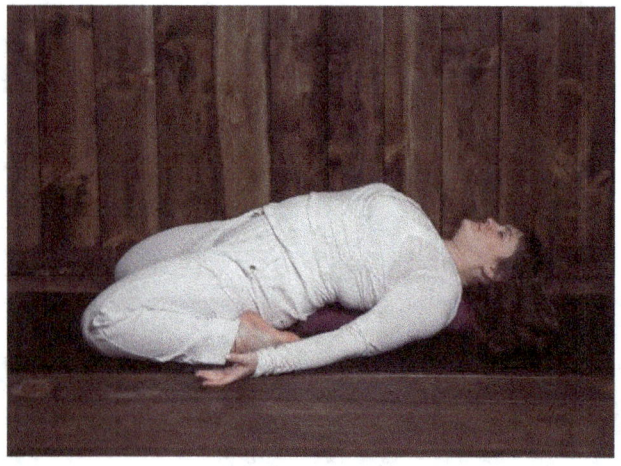

- Modification: support your body with a bolster

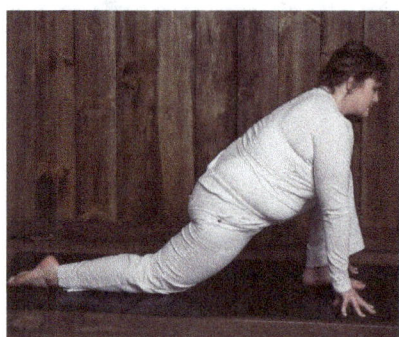 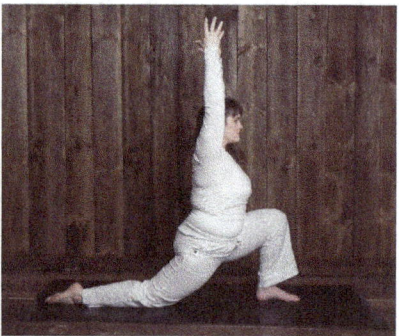

Low Lunge (Anjaneyasana): Either from Table Pose or Downward Dog, step the right foot between your hands (knee above ankle) and drop the left knee to the mat. Keep your hips square and as you scoot your hips forward and allow them to drop toward the ground, find the comfortable edge of those pose in your body (i.e., you can hold the pose and breathe, but you feel it's a little challenge).

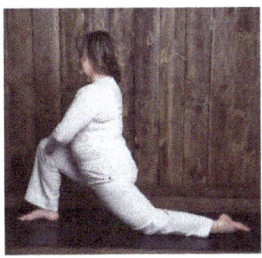 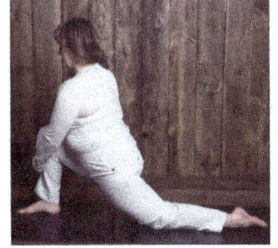 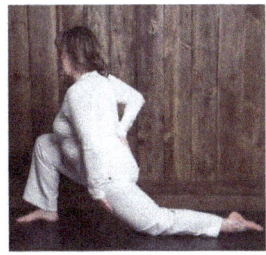

Low lunge variations with Reiki hand positions

- Hands can be on the ground/blocks, thighs, or hips, depending on the torso position.
- You can give yourself an intuitive hand position. Helpful hand positions here include: heart, low belly, groin/hips, thighs and glutes, lower back.

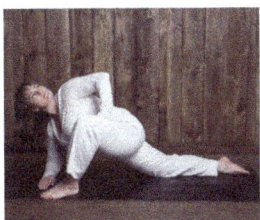 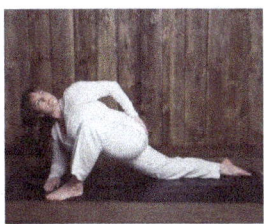 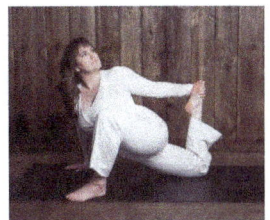

Lizard pose with Reiki hand positions, and a quad stretch variation

- To explore the hip mobility, and for more experienced yogi(ni)s, it's an option to take a variation of **Lizard Pose (Utthan Pristhasana)**. Walk out the front foot to about 45 degrees (toes pointing to the outside corner of the mat, opening happens from the hip, not the knee), and lower your torso closer to the ground, to a level that is sustainable (i.e. a comfortable edge where you are still breathing normally).
- Do the other side.

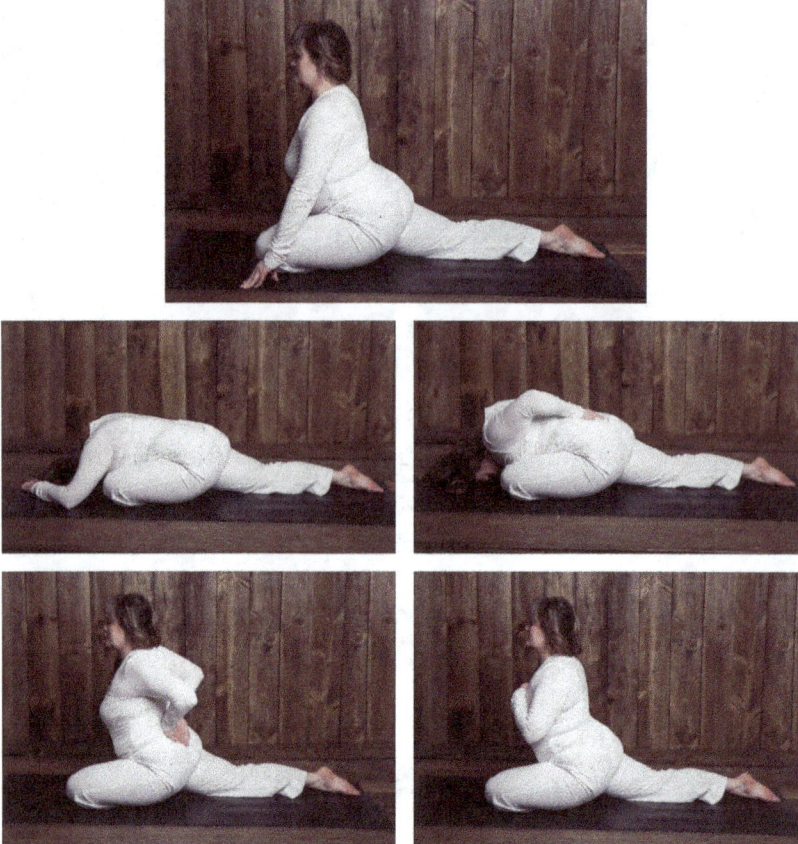

Pigeon (or swan) with forward fold option, and Reiki hand positions

Pigeon Pose (Kapotasana): Either from downward dog or table pose, send your right knee to your right wrist, allowing your shin to point at 7 o'clock (in a 45-degree angle). Keep your pelvis square (i.e., both hips are facing forward) and lower your pelvis to the ground as is comfortable, keeping low-back sensitivity in mind! Tip: Place a block or bolster under the right hip/glutes to keep the hips square and to control the intensity of the pose.

- Once in (upward) Pigeon Pose, you may choose to stay for several breaths, or hold for a few breaths before offering yourself a forward fold into resting Pigeon.
- Many stretching options are possible from pigeon, whether you wish to focus on more extensions or lateral stretches. Feel free to explore!
- If traditional Pigeon pose is not comfortable, namely due to knee injuries, you can modify by doing the pose in seated "staff" position and creating figure-four stretches onto each thigh, or taking the supine figure-four stretch (onto your back). Pigeon can also be done on a chair!
- Do the other side (i.e., left knee to left wrist, shin and toes pointing at 5 o'clock, sliding the block under the left hip/glutes)
- *Traditional Pigeon Pose is another great opportunity for Reiki yoga teachers to provide hands-on assists.*
- *If you choose a pigeon modification, you may find yourself in a position to offer yourself a Reiki treatment.*

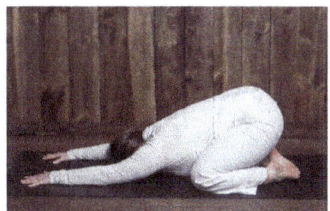

Child's Pose (Balasana): Resume Child's Pose, by sending your hips back to your heels and folding forward, toward your thighs. Arms can be forward or by your body.

- Child's Pose is not favourable for self-treatments, but is a great opportunity for Reiki yoga teacher to offer a hands-on Reiki yoga assist.

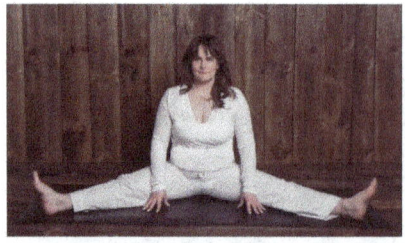
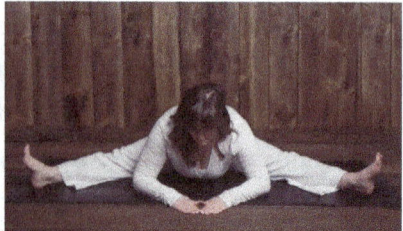
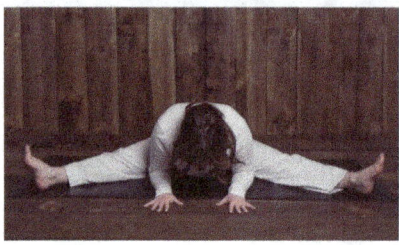

Wide leg straddle with forward fold variations; blocks of bolsters can also be used to support the upper body for a more restorative practice.

Wide Leg Straddle (V): Sitting upright (grounded from sitz bones, neutral pelvis, back in axial extension), open your legs into a wide V shape (i.e., dragonfly pose in yin yoga) and keep a gentle bend in the knees (do not lock articulations).

- You may take side bends, and/or fold onto each leg. These poses also allow for self-treatments, provided you can comfortably reach the body part you wish to assist.
- While keeping the pelvis neutral and grounded, fold from the hip crease into a forward fold. This can be a few inches and still be effective, it's not about reaching any destination.
- If needed, bend one leg into a **Half Dragonfly**, prop your pelvis up with a folded blanket or bolster, and/or roll up blankets to place under the knees.
- For advanced yogi(ni)s, or for those whose mobility allows and feels good to do so, there's an option to take

Turtle Pose (Kurmasana), by folding forward and sliding arms under the legs (palms down).

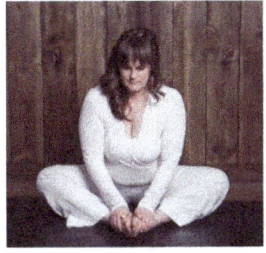 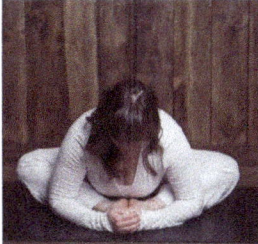 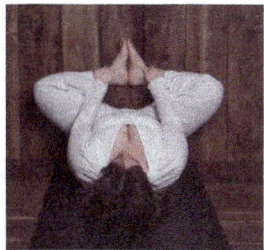

Butterfly pose, with options for forward fold, or use a wall

Butterfly Pose (Titli Asana) or Reclined Butterfly: From your wide V, bring the soles of your feet together for butterfly pose for a few breaths.

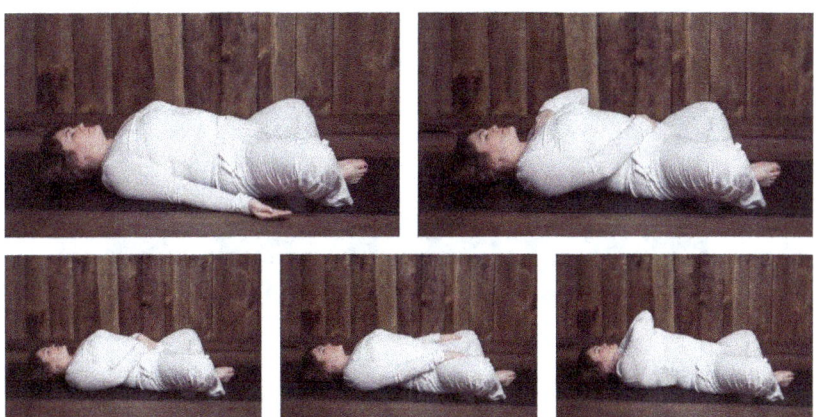

Reclined butterfly with optional Reiki hand positions

- You can then assist the knees together, lie down, and resume in reclined butterfly (i.e., on your back). Feel free to use blocks or a bolster to support the knees and thighs here.

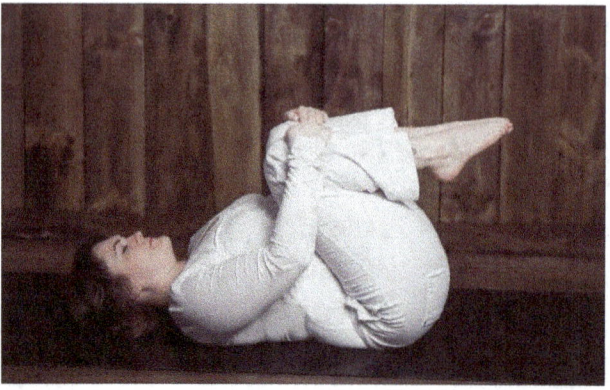

- Assist your legs back to centre, and **hug knees into your chest (apanasana)**.

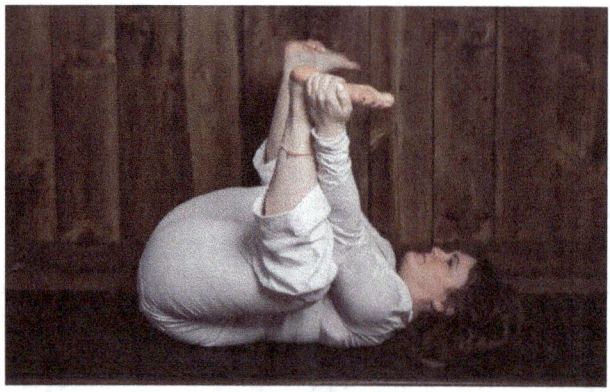

Happy Baby Pose (Ananda Balasana): hugging your knees into your chest, open your legs from the hip, intending your knees toward your armpits. Grab the outside of your feet (or grab the big toes between thumb and index and middle fingers), and press your soles toward the sky. It is like your squatting in the air! Release after a few deep breaths.

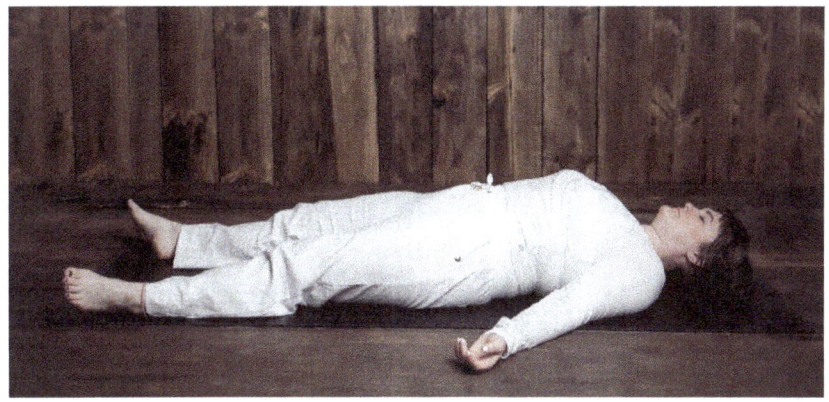

Savasana: Lie on your back, palms up/shoulder blades down to allow the long neck, adding any props or support your need.

USUI REIKI MANTRA OPTION: Cho Ku Rei

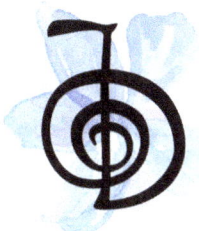

Drawn traditionally or chanted in crescendo, Cho Ku Rei increases power, physical strength, vitality.

Drawn in reverse or chanted in decrescendo, Cho Ku Rei can also be used to decrease the intensity of a less desirable condition, disease/illness, symptom or feeling.

YOGA MEDITATION OPTIONS:

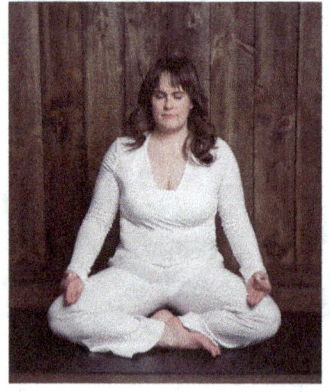

Om mani padme hum mantra (clears all negative energy) with chin / gyan mudra

Shiva linga mudra (efficient energy use): left hand over the navel area is held in a soft cupping, right hand forms a fist with your thumb sticking up. Place the right hand into the left to increase the efficiency of energy.

Energizing breaths (like breath of fire, kapalabhati, or any kundalini immune meditation)

Ujjayi (aka ocean breath)

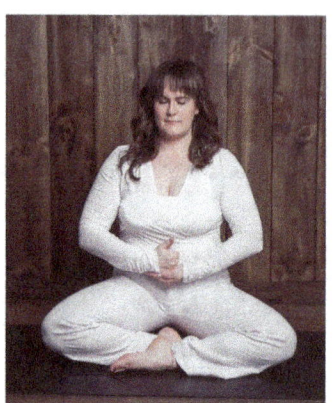

SEQUENCE 2: FEELING
PRACTICE FOCUS BY AREA: BACK & TORSO

THIS SEQUENCE ACTIVATES and balances lower and central chakras, which include the sacral, solar plexus, and heart chakras. These chakras deal primarily with our emotional body, hence the theme of "feeling." For simplicity's sake, I will call the traditional heart chakra the "heart." I will refer only briefly to the combination of what advanced reiki practitioners may refer to as the triad of heart chakras often called the "etheric heart" of universal love and compassion, which include the traditional heart chakra, the ascending heart and the sacred heart. I personally like to call it the "Great Heart" which to me, includes all three.

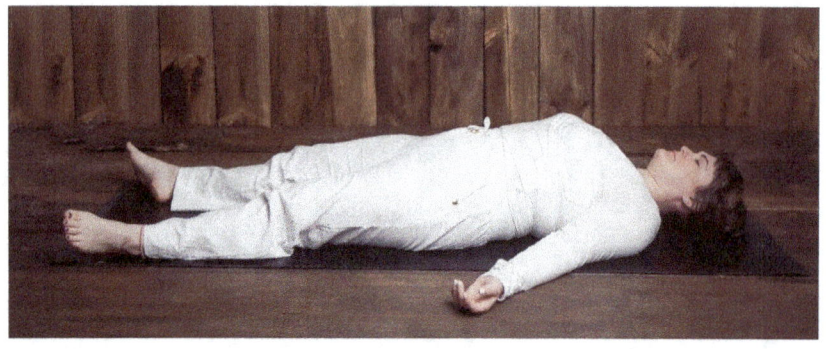

Savasana: lie on your back comfortably.

Reiki Meditation: activate the flow of Reiki within with the breath and visualization previously described.

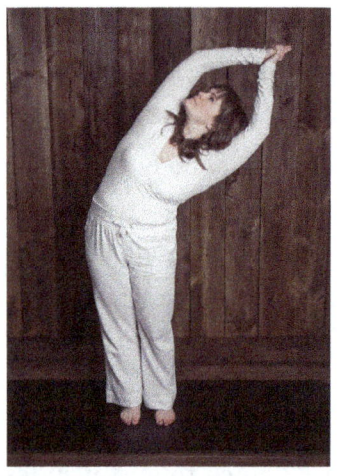

Shown standing up as Half-Moon Stretch, but Bananasana is a supine pose. Ankles can be crossed, opposite elbows or hands can be held for additional stretch.

Banana Stretch (Bananasana): To get into this lateral stretch, lie on back with arms overhead. Walk your arms to the right top corner of your mat. You can hook wrists or elbows here for stability and additional stretch. Keeping your back and hips flat and grounded, walk your feet to the bottom right corner of your mat. You can cross your ankles for stability. You body is now forming a banana-like shape, as you create length in your side body. This is not a twist!

- You may want to pause on your back between sides to assess how your body is interacting with the pose.
- Do the other side.

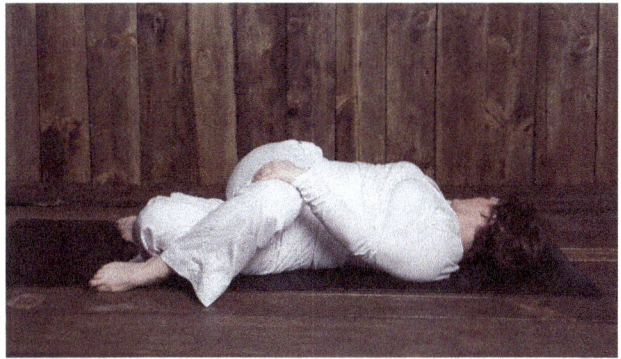

Reclined Twists: Lying on your back, feet flat on the mat, move your hips to the right of your mat and send your knees to the left. Your arms can rest by your side, or in a "T" shape.

You can place a hand on your heart and one on your lower back for self-treatment, or simply breathe into this pose.

- You can choose to cross your legs (right over left on this side).
- Do the other side.

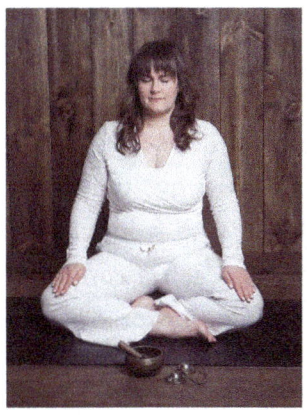
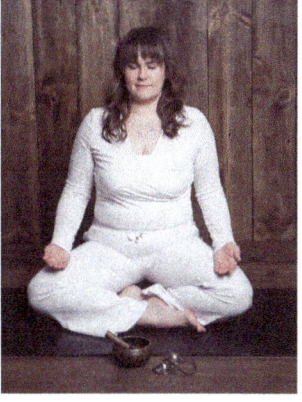

Easy Pose (Sukhasana): From lying on your back, hug your knees into your chest and give yourself a gentle rock side to side, and begin to rock back and forth. You can either build momentum to come to seated, or turn to your side and use your arms to help yourself into an easy seat, legs crossed (with or without blocks to support the knees, or a blanket/bolster to prop the pelvis into a neutral position). Palms face down for grounding, or up for energy.

- Scan your body and practice a self-treatment. Focus on the top of your body and on the back.

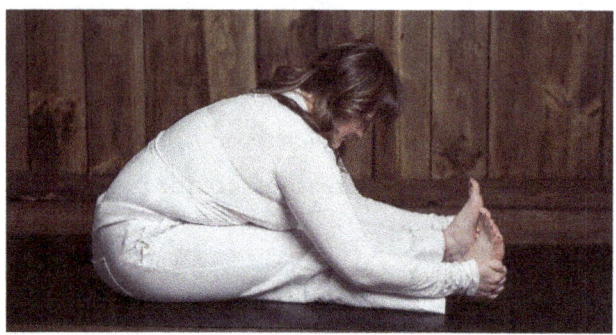

West Stretch (Paschimottanasana): From a sitting position (neutral pelvis means you are sitting on your sitz bones), extend your legs forward, don't lock your knees, and feel free to slide a rolled blanket under your knees to relieve pressure from your hamstrings or lower back. Inhale to grow tall (i.e., an axial extension of your spine), and fold forward from your hip crease (not from the waist); stop when you reach a comfortable edge. Take a few breaths here. Exhale to bring your torso back up.

- Practice the lower body self-treatment, focusing on legs and feet. You can bend each leg into a figure-four shape to facilitate.

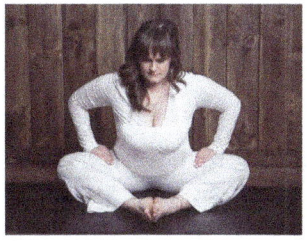 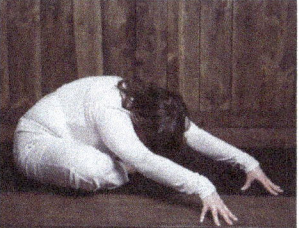

Butterfly (Titli Asana): From sitting, bring the soles of your feet together, and adjust your feet closer or farther away from you, depending on what feels better for you. Inhale to grow tall, exhale to fold forward from your hip crease. Hold the pose for two to four breaths.

- Option to hold the fold in butterfly, and walk hands to each corner of the mat, taking a few breaths on each side, to provide an additional lower back stretch.

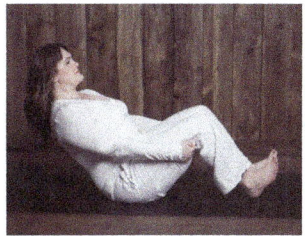 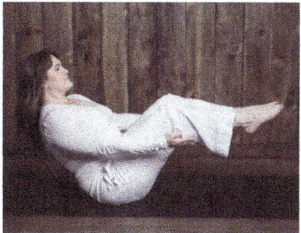

Boat Pose (Navasana): if you are looking to fire up the abdominals (and the solar plexus chakra), root your sitz bones down, extend your spine tall, feet on the ground. You can lean back to a 45-degree angle.

- You can hold onto the back of your thighs and keep your heels on the mat for a gentler, beginner-friendly version.

- You can choose to lift your feet up and reach our arms forward for a challenge.
- Experienced yogi(ni)s may choose a more challenging version, if they can maintain posture integrity of a neutral pelvis and extended spine. They would extend both arms and legs up, forming a "V" shape with your profile.

Reversed Table Pose (Urdhva Bharmanasana): Feet flat on the mat, hip-distance apart, hands are slightly wider than shoulder width apart behind you, fingers pointing toward your hips. Press up on all fours, sending your hips, belly, and heart to the sky. Hold for two to four breaths.

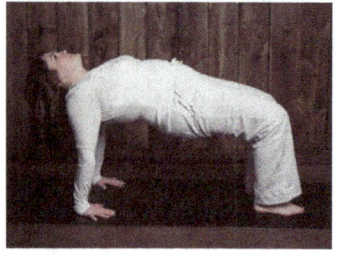

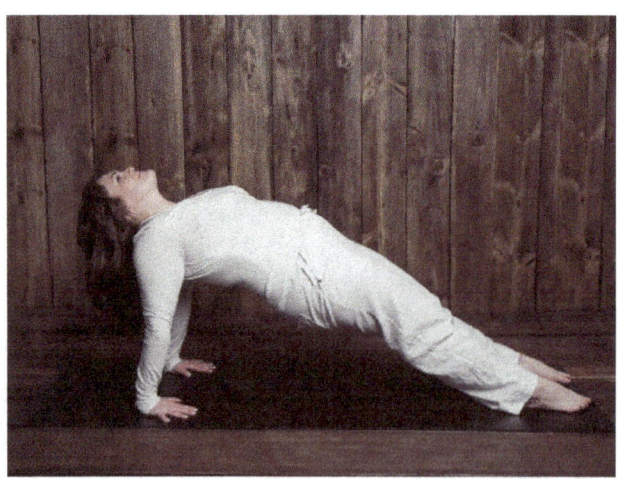

- Modification to engage abdominals, take **Upward Plank Pose (Purvottanasana)**. Press up with legs extended forward instead of bent knees.

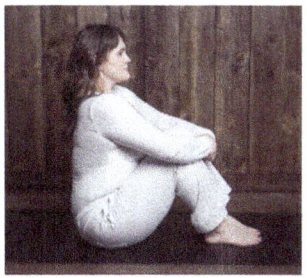 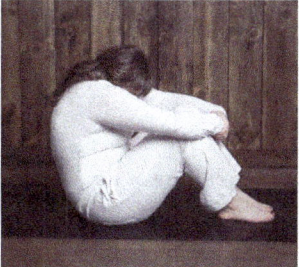

- Option to take a **Seated Cat-Cow**. Inhale to grow tall, hugging the knees into your chest; exhale round out your back.

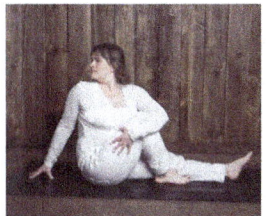 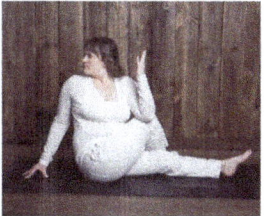 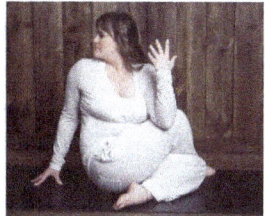

Left to right, Half Lord of the Fishes twist options for varying degrees of hip and back mobility.

Seated Twist or Half Lord of the Fishes (Ardha Matsyendrasana): From seated, hug the right knee into your chest, wrap the right leg with your left arm, and twist to the right, while sitting tall. Do the other side.

- Experienced yogi(ni)s may wish to modify this into Half Lord of the Fishes twist (Ardha Matsyendrasana): hug the right knee to your chest, cross right foot over left leg, inhale to grow tall and reach up with left arm, twist to the right and let the left elbow rest on the outside of the right thigh, as you sit tall. Lastly, wrap the right leg to the left, as if to sit cross-legged. Do the other side.

- Reminder: do the other side of your chosen twist!

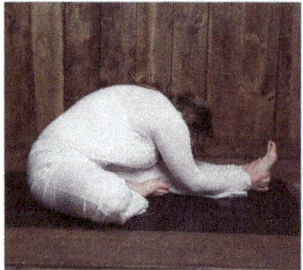
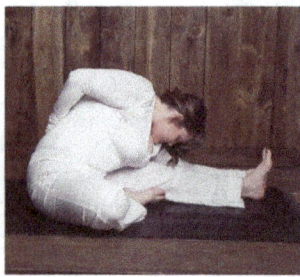

- Option to take **Knee-to-Nose Pose (Janu Sirsasana)**: from seated, extend the left leg forward, bring the right sole to the inside of the left thigh. Inhale to grow tall, exhale to fold forward from the hip crease. After a few breaths, you may choose to add a gentle extension by placing the right hand behind your right hip, and pressing down, lifting your hips up, reaching the left arm overhead into a lateral stretch. Do the other side.

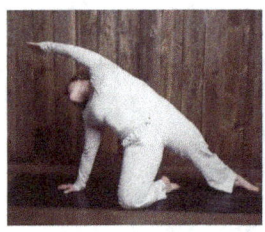
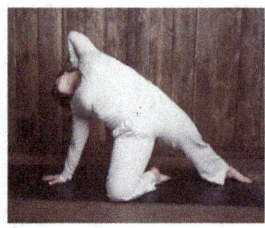
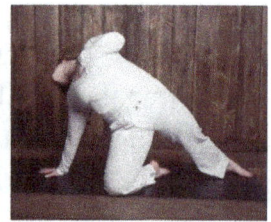

Option to take a brief extension into a **Supported Side Plank (Vasisthasana)**. Place the right hand outside your right hip, and press through your right hand and left foot, lifting your hips and stretching your left side body. You can use your left hand to offer Reiki intuitively. Do the other side.

To add a dynamic portion when your body and energy call for it, add this mini sequence here. Otherwise, resume at the Three-Legged Dog below.

Sun Salutation

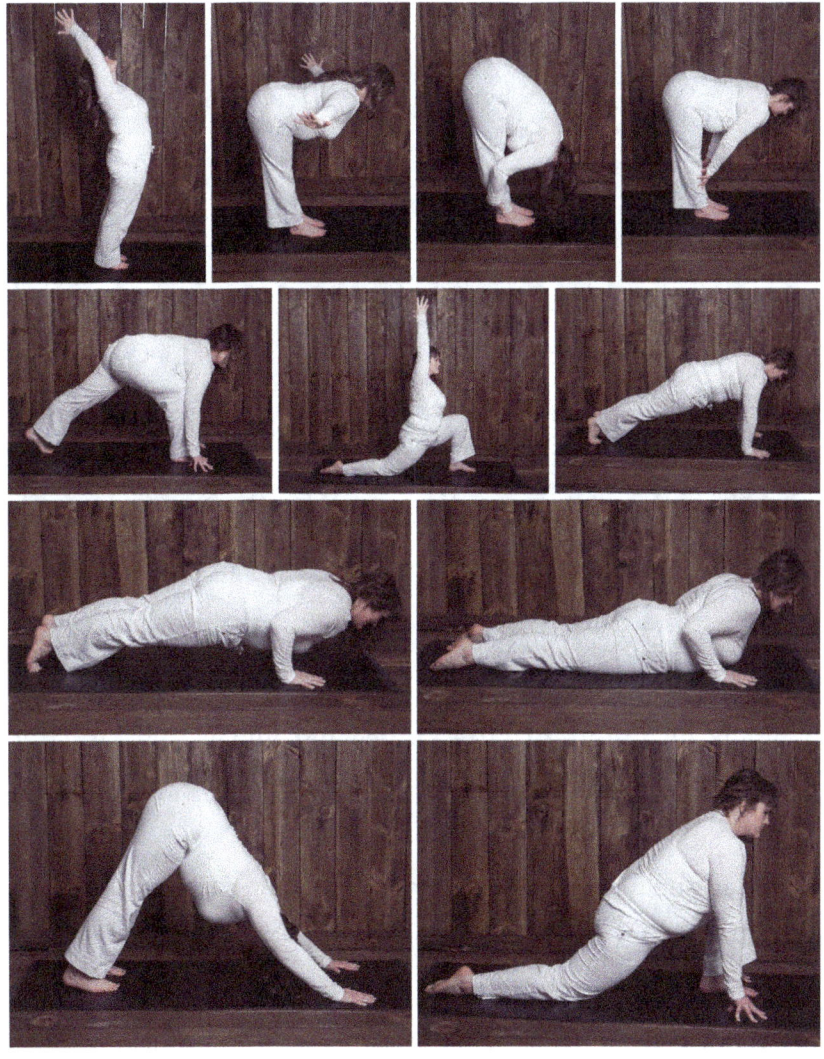

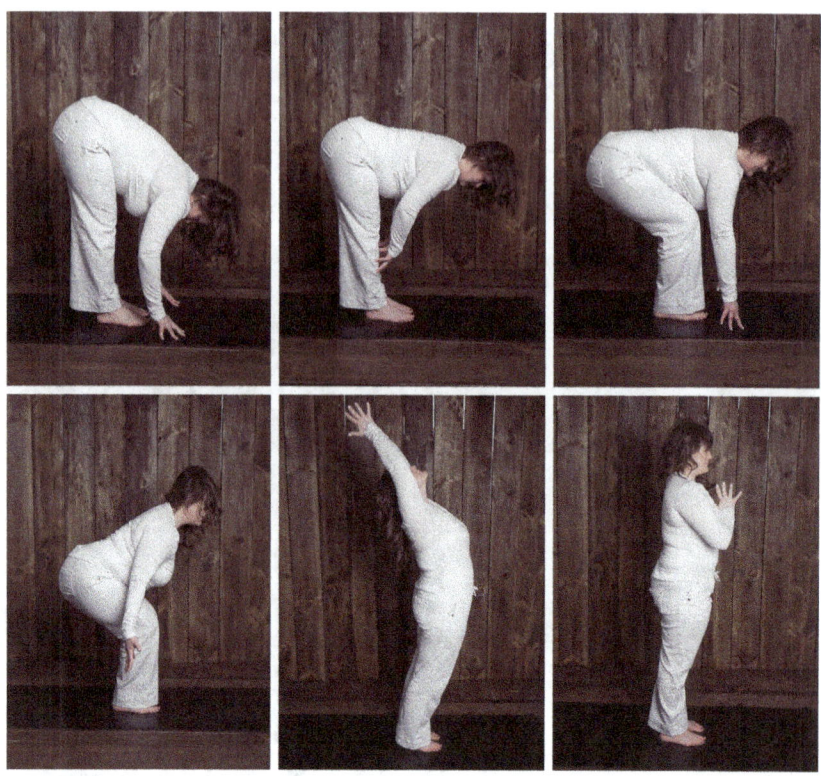

Practice one round of a Classic Sun Salutation (Surya Namaskara):

Standing in **Mountain Pose (Tadasana)**, inhale your arms up overhead (from the front instead of the sides if there are shoulder injuries), exhale **fold forward (Uttanasana)**.

Inhale lift halfway, exhale step your left foot back into a **Lunge (Anjaneyasana)**, inhale into your lunge.

Exhale, step the right foot back (together), inhale in your **Plank (Phalakasana)** and rock your heels forward if you choose to be on your feet (instead of your knees), exhale **lower your body to the ground (Chaturanga)**.

Inhale pull the top of your head forward, draw your shoulder blades down your back, keep your neck long and lift your heart into your version of **Cobra (Baby Cobra, Full Cobra, or even the challenging Upward Dog** if you have the abdominal strength and your low back is not stressed).

Exhale into **Downward Dog (Adho Mukha Svanasana)**; you may transition through table to get to Downward Dog as this is gentler on the back is the abdominal strength is not present to sustain this transition. Step the left foot forward to lunge on the other side. Inhale in your lunge. Exhale your feet together at the top of your mat into a **forward fold**.

Inhale into a **half lift (Ardha Uttanasana)**, exhale fold once more. Bend your knees and send your hips back as though about to sit, lengthen your spine and neck, and inhale yourself up to standing by pressing through your legs. Take a gentle backbend if it feels good. Exhale hands to your heart, in Anjali Mudra (prayer or salutation mudra).

<u>Repeat, but this time you begin by stepping the right foot back into your lunge, and stepping it forward to complete your salutation.</u>

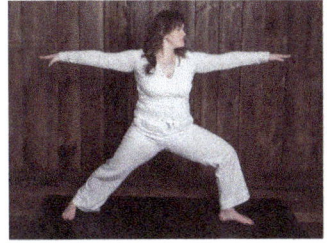
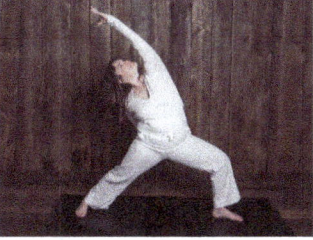
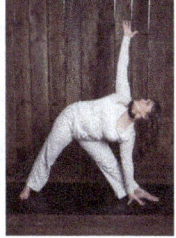

Warrior II (Virabhadrasana II), Exalted Warrior (Viparita Virabhadrasana) and Triangle pose (Trikonasana) mini flow.

Warrior II:

Step the left foot back into a lunge, then turn your heel in at a 90-degree angle (i.e., your front (right) heel lines up perfectly with your back arch [left foot]). Your hips are slightly off the front, facing 10 o'clock instead. Your right knee is directly above your right ankle and if your alignment is safe, you cannot see your right big toe (if you can see it, your knee is dipping inside your hip line, which strains your knee—perhaps shorten your stance to maintain a better alignment). Extend your arms out and gaze forward for a few breaths. *(Keep in mind, you'll have to do the other side of this pose at the end of your mini sequence.)*

Exalted warrior:

On an exhale breath, lengthen your spine up and raw your right arm and gaze to the sky, dropping the left arm toward your left thigh (or left the top of your hand rest on the lower back). If your neck is sensitive, look down toward your left calf. Hold Exalted Warrior for a few breaths. *(Keep in mind, you'll have to do the other side of this pose at the end of your mini sequence)*

Triangle pose:

On an inhale breath, return to Warrior II. Lengthen the right light, sway your hips to the back of your mat (in this example, toward the left hip), reach forward to the top of your mat, then fold from your hip crease (not your waist!) into a lateral fold, effectively creating triangle pose. You can rest your right hand on a block, on your thigh or your shin if that is more comfortable or accessible to you than the mat directly. Your left arm can stay up, or your hand can come rest on your left hip, or the top of your hand on your low back for a slight rotation of the shoulder. *(Keep in mind, you'll have to do the other side of this pose at the end of your mini sequence)*

Advanced Option: You can choose to incorporate these three poses into the previous sun salutation, or add two rounds of said salutation and replace the lunge portion with the Warrior II, Exalted Warrior, and Triangle Mini Flow.

Do both sides.

Resume here if you skipped the dynamic portion.

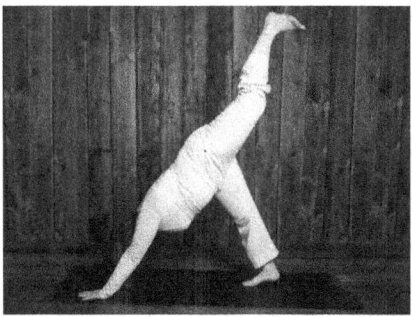

Three-Legged Dog: From table pose, press into Downward Dog. Place your right foot toward the middle line of the mat, creating a tripod between your hands and foot. Keeping your hips square (i.e., facing the ground), lift your left leg up into Three-Legged Dog.

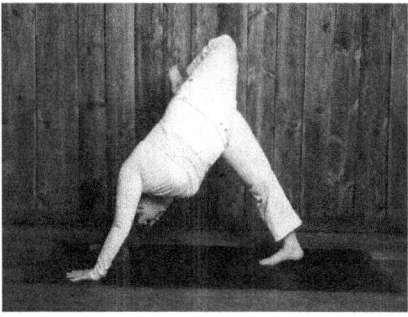

- Bend your right knee and send your heel over your left hip, to open the hips and get a bit of an oblique stretch.

- Do the other side.

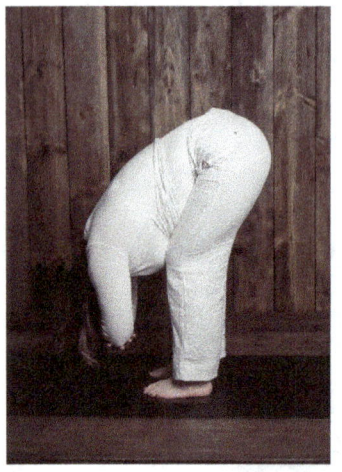

Rag Doll: Step the feet together at the top of your mat, bend the knees deeply, and allow your back, neck and head to hang with gravity. Let your arms fall or hook opposite elbows. You can also interlace fingers behind your head for additional neck stretch, if that feels good to you. After a few breaths, take a wide stance and lower your hips onto a deep squat, Garland Pose (Malasana).

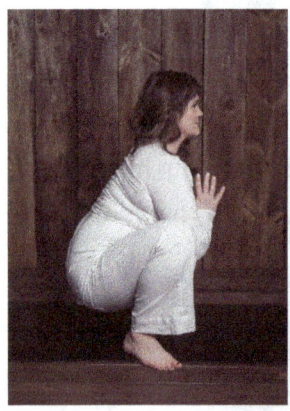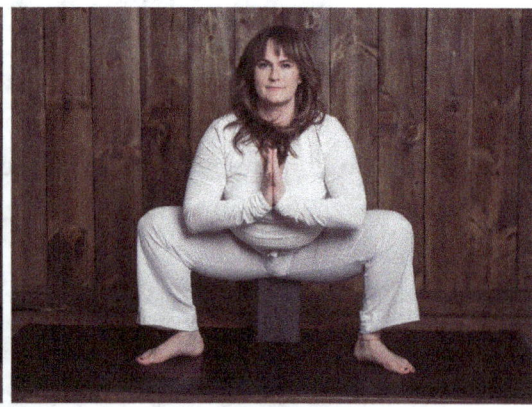

Garland Pose (Malasana): Squat deeply, with feet wider than hip distance apart, preferably with a gentle outward 45-degree angle to your feet (as long as your knees point in the same direction as your toes!). You may use a block for support to sit on. Hold this squat for a few breaths.

Come out of the squat, and find your way onto your back.

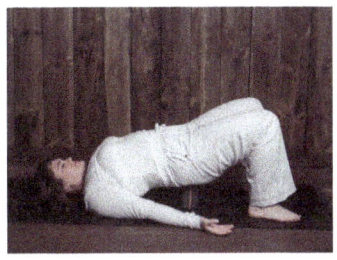

Supported Bridge (Setu Bandha Sarvangasana): Feet flat on the mat, lift your hips, and slide a block or bolster under your sacrum (i.e., the bony triangle between your glutes and your lumbar spine), let your hips rest on the support. Arms can rest by your side or overhead (on the ground).

- Option to take **Supported Waterfall Pose**, by lifting the legs to the sky (gentle bend in the knees). You may wish to place your hands intuitively on your body, or simply be in the pose.

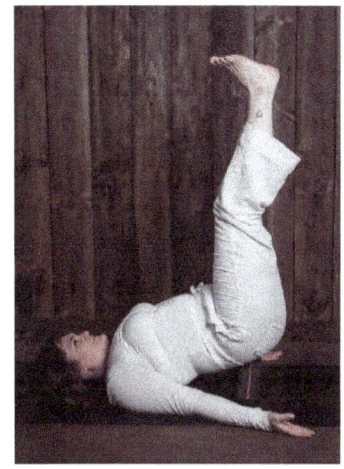

- Advanced option: If it is safe for you and in your practice, you may wish to take **Shoulder Stand (Salamba Sarvangasana)** by placing your hands on the hips, keeping the neck neutral once you lift the hips, and extend the legs to the sky. You may want to use the hands' natural supportive placement as a self-treatment opportunity.

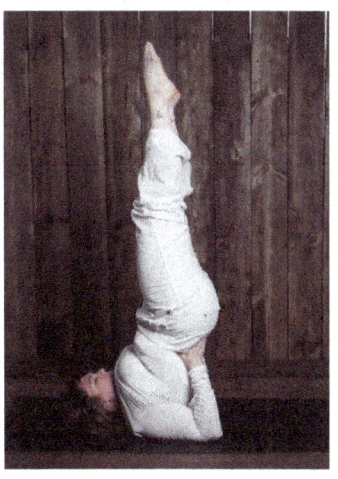

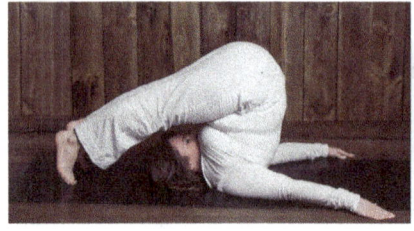 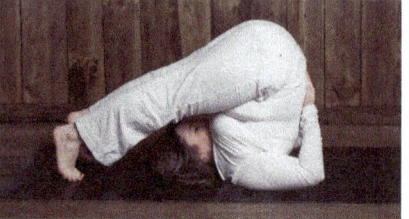

- Additional advanced option to take **Plow Pose (Halasana)**, by sending the feet overhead towards the ground (from Shoulder Sand), if that feels good for you.
- Come out of your chosen pose and variation on your exhale and take a few moments to allow the spine to shift back to neutral position.

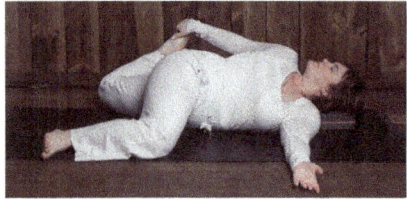 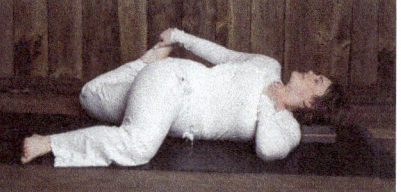

Cat Pulling Its Tail: Lying on your stomach, prop your torso onto your forearms (i.e. sphinx pose) and bring your right knee out to your right side in a 90-degree angle, keeping your shin parallel to your left leg. It may look like you are climbing. Press your right hand into the ground, slide your left hand (palm facing up) under your right arm and drop your left shoulder down. Rest your head on the ground or on a block to support the neck. Bend your left leg and reach for your foot with your right hand (you may use a strap).

- You can simply rest in this pose, or add hands intuitively.
- Do the other side.

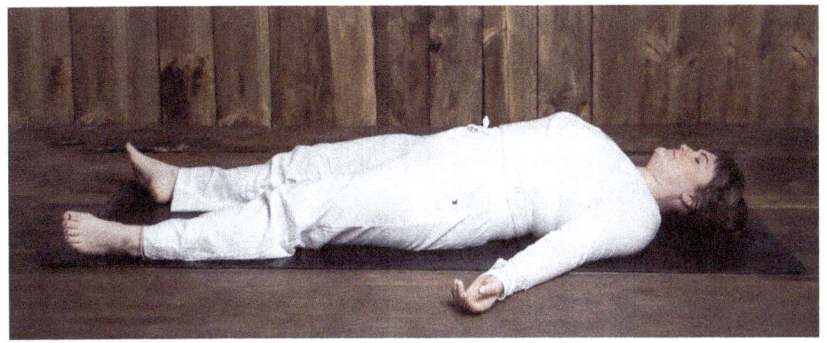

Savasana (integration/final meditation): lie on your back comfortably.

USUI REIKI MANTRA OPTION: Sei Hei Ki

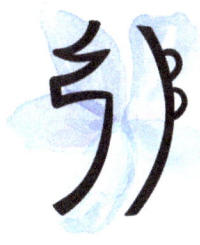

Sei Hei Ki is a useful symbol for emotional clearing and empowerment.

As a mantra, it can be used to restore a calm, peaceful heart, gain perspective and detach from outcomes.

YOGA MEDITATION OPTIONS:

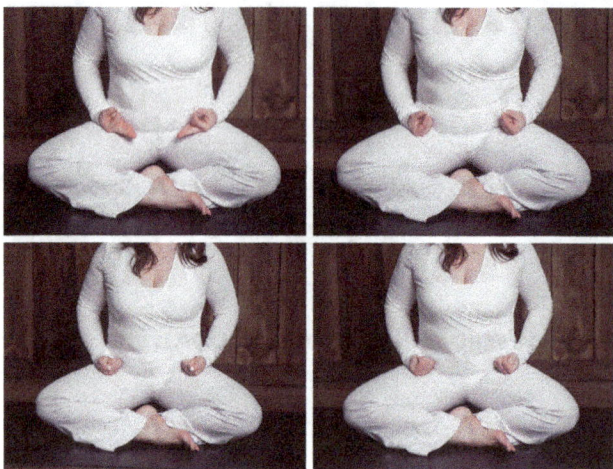

- **Yoga breath with mudras:** This breath helps guide the breath to use the full lung capacity with practice, over time.
- In seated position, place your hands on the hip crease in chin / Gyan Mudra (index and thumb). Then keep the index/thumb together and wrap the other fingers into a fist. For your third mudra, form a fist with your thumb resting just on the outside, leaning up against the side of the index. Lastly, wrap your thumb with all your fingers.
- Take 4-8 breaths with each mudra

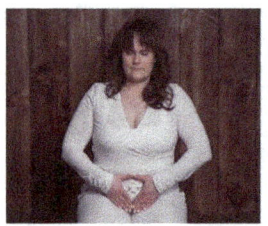 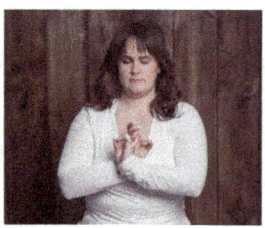 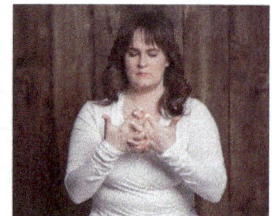

- **Trimurti Mudra** ("three forms", for transitions), **Fearless Heart Mudra** (Abhaya Hridaya), OR **Unshakable Trust Mudra** (Vajrapradama)

SEQUENCE 3: OPENING/LIGHTENING/ EXPANDING
PRACTICE FOCUS BY AREA: HEAD, NECK, & SHOULDERS

THIS SEQUENCE ACTIVATES and balances the upper chakras, as well as the heart and Great Heart. The upper chakras include the throat, third eye, crown and soul chakras. The soul chakra is located about a foot or 30 cm above the crown and top of the head, and connects us to our soul (the part of us that incarnates and retains memory), oneness and the divine, which is to say our spirit and the Great Spirit/Universe/God/Goddess. It is also an energy portal to what shamanic traditions call the Upper World.

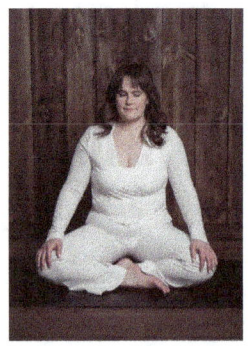

Seated Comfortably (Sukhasana): sit comfortably, with sitz bones grounded, pelvis neutral (i.e., back is not arched or rounded), back in axial extension (i.e., growing tall), neck is long (i.e., chin is tucked back gently, not down).

Reiki meditation: activate the flow of Reiki energy with the breath and visualization described previously.

Body scan: Using cupped hands hovering a few inches above/away from your physical body, scan yourself from head to toe.

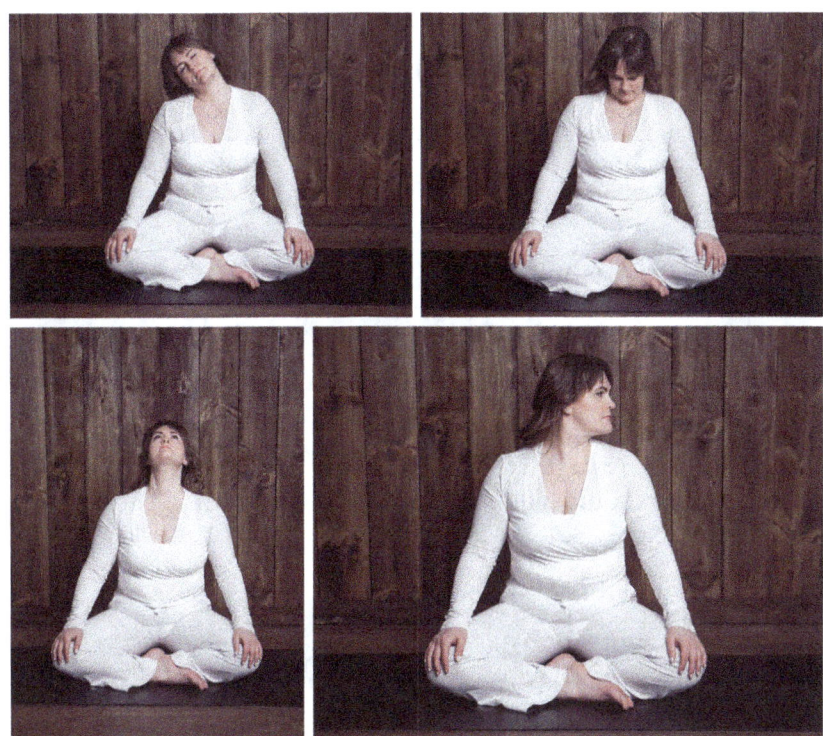

Head and shoulder movements:

- Look to both sides, then up and down, following your breath.
- Rock your head softly side to side, sending one ear toward the shoulder then the other.

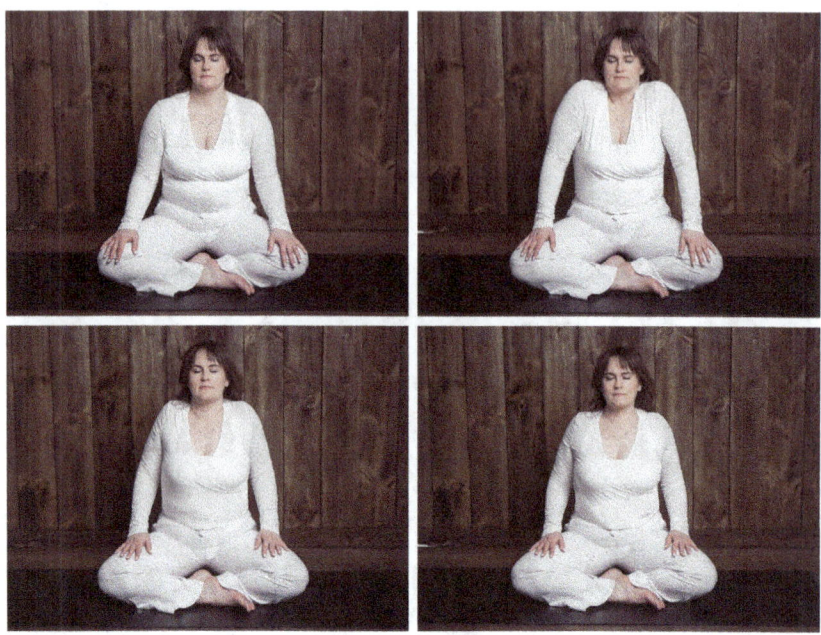

- Roll your shoulders front for a few breaths, then back.
- Lift your shoulders up on the inhale, exhale drop them. Repeat a few times as needed.

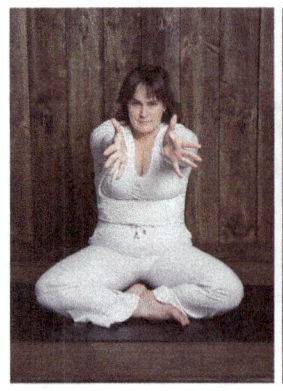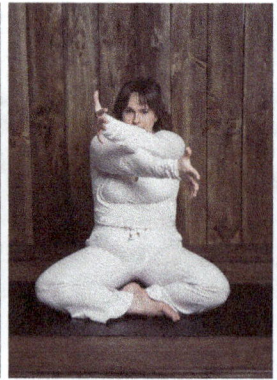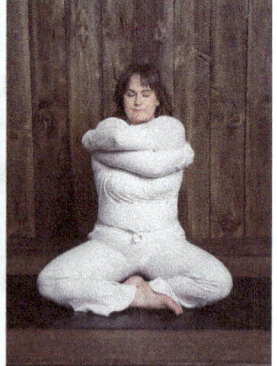

WING MOVEMENTS:

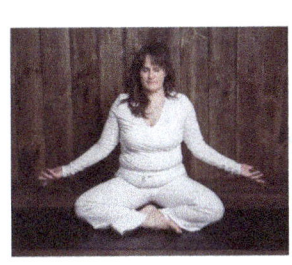 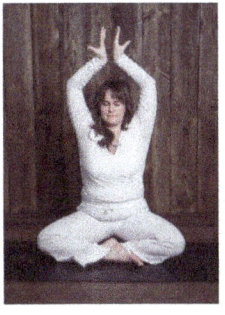 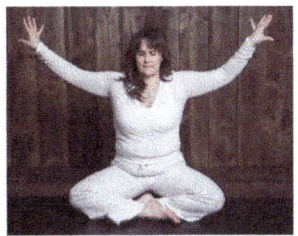

- Inhale your arms up beside you palms up, exhale press your arms down with resistance, palms down.

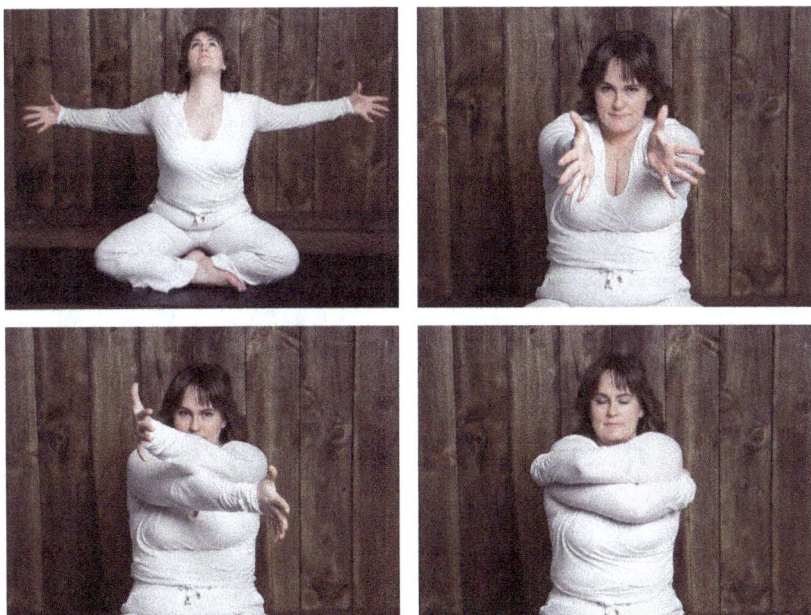

- Inhale open your arms wide, open your heart, look up; exhale bring your palms back together flapping the wings closed, rounding out your back, allowing your head to gently curl in. Repeat for a few breaths.

- On your next exhale, wrap your wings by crossing your arms and reaching for opposite scapulas (i.e., shoulder blades). Extend your spine up, neck is long/chin neutral, play around with the height of your elbows here. Do the other side (i.e., cross the other arm on top).

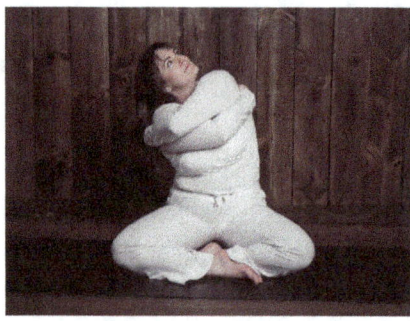

- Option: Engage your abdominals and take side bends, for a few breaths on each side, and use your exhale to return to centre.

Eagle Arms + Cow Face Arms:

- **Eagle Arms:** wrap the right arm under the left, and hook your hands, hold for a few breaths. Wrap the left arm under the right to do the other side.

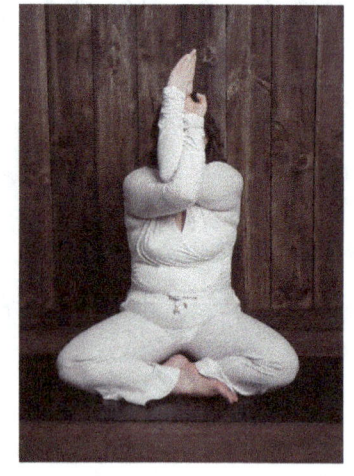

Modification: Simply bring (or intend) the forearms and palms together; elbows are about shoulder height.

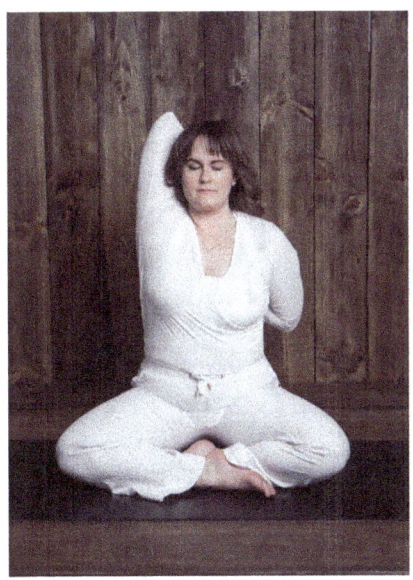 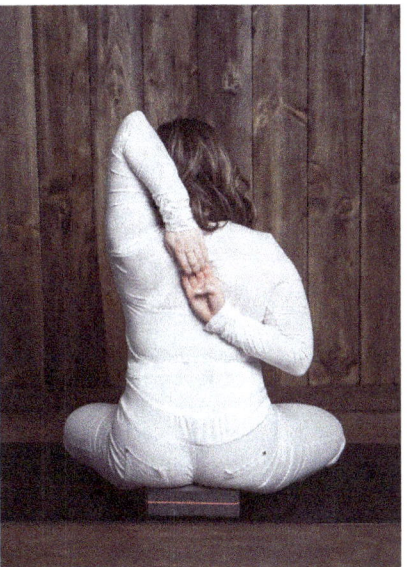

Cow Face Arms: reach up with your right arm and place fingers between scapulas. Turn the left thumb inward, bend the elbow and reach for the right hand (or strap!). To do the other side, reach up with the left arm, bend the elbow and place the fingers between the scapulas. Turn the right thumb in, bend the elbow and reach for the left hand (or strap).

- If mobility is an issue, don't hesitate to use a yoga strap, towel or soft belt as a tool.
- Modification: If there's a shoulder injury, a modification would be to simply place the palm of the hand behind the head and the back of the other hand on the low back.
- These arm poses are opportunities for Reiki assists and yoga adjustments from experienced instructors.

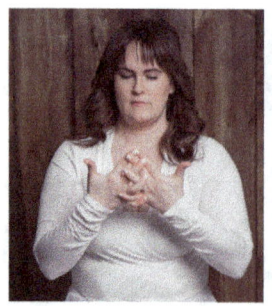 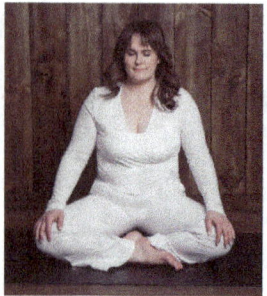 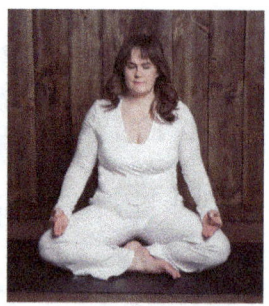

Hand/wrist movements:

- Roll your wrists in both directions for a few breaths.
- Hold out one hand, palm up, and using the other hand, stretch the palm open/down. Then gently press each finger back slightly. Do both hands.
- Interlace your fingers together and trace a figure eight with your knuckles. Do the other direction.
- From the top of the hand, gently press, sending the palm toward the forearm, stretching the top of the wrist—carefully! Do both hands.

Top body hand positions:

- focus on your head, neck, shoulders, and arms

TORSO MOVEMENTS:

- **Seated Twists**: from a seated position (neutral pelvis rooted down, extended spine), inhale centre, exhale turn your torso to the right and hold for a few breaths. Hands can be on the outside of your opposite thigh and one behind you. Do the twist on the left side.

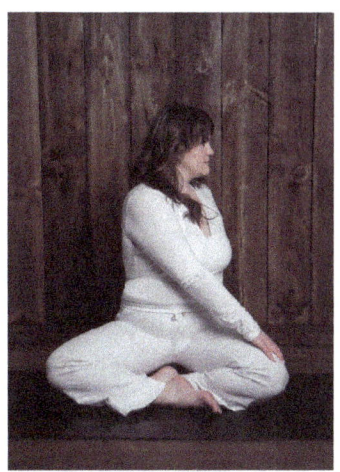

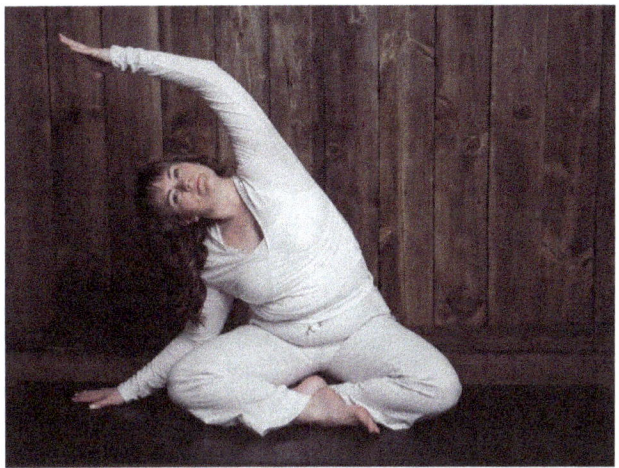

- **Side bends**: from a seated position (as above), place the right hand on the mat beside you, reach up with your left arm on the inhale, exhale reach to the right into a side bend and hold for a few breaths. Do the other side, by placing the left hand beside you, reaching the right arm up on the inhale, exhale to reach over to the left, holding in a side bend for a few breaths.

Table (Bharmanasana): On all fours, place hands under shoulders, fingers spread and engaged to ease the pressure in the wrists. Knees are under hips, pelvis is neutral (no arching, no rounding of the back). The back looks like a table top.

- **Cat-Cow**: Inhale drop the belly and softly arm your back as is comfortable, exhale tuck your navel in and round your back. Follow this movement for a few breaths.
- **Barrel Roll**: this is an option if you'd like to explore movement with your rib cage. Draw circles with your torso by bringing your heart toward the mat on the inhale, and exhale complete the circle by coming up and rounding out your back. Draw circles in both directions for balance.

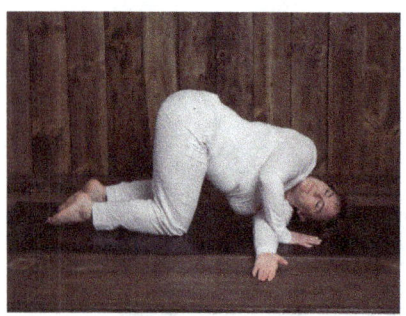 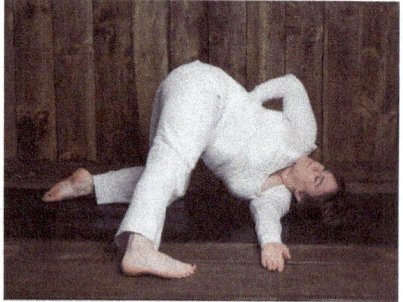

Thread the Needle (Parsva Balasana):

- From all fours (table pose), scoop the right hand under your left arm, palm up, and place your shoulder on the mat. You can support your head with a blanket or block to make this more comfortable. Do the other side: scoop your left hand under your right arm, palm up, placing the left shoulder down, and supporting

- Option to take this into a **Gate Pose (Parighasana) variation**: from all fours, extend your right foot straight out beside you, toes forward, foot flat. Scoop the right hand under the left arm palm up. For the other side, extend the left leg out, and scoop the left hand under thee right arm, palm up.

Child's Pose (Balasana): send your hips back toward your heels and fold forward. Arms can be extended forward or resting by your side.

- There's an opportunity for Reiki assist by a teacher or facilitator: hands can be placed on the back and/or hips, with permission from the student/client.

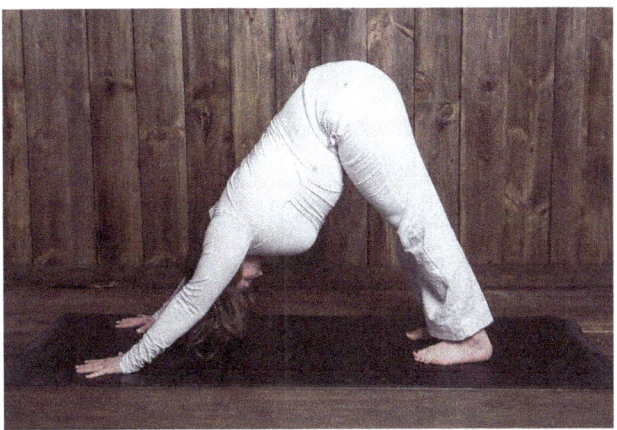

Downward Dog (Adho Mukha Svanasana): Slightly wider than shoulder width apart, fingers spread wide, press through your hands and finger pads, curl your toes under and send your hips back and up, forming an A shape.

- Focus on the length of your spine from a neutral pelvis (no rounding, no arching). Tip: You may want to keep heels off the floor for a while, and keep a more pronounced bend in the knees (never lock the knees anyway!) until both the back of the thighs (hamstrings) and lower back can comfortably accommodate the deeper stretch associated with an extended leg. Heels may approach the ground with practice, but they may not either. The pose is still the pose, whether the heels ground or not.

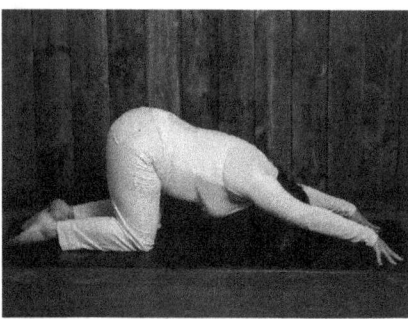

- <u>Modification:</u> You may choose to take **Puppy Stretch**, which is the same pose, but on your knees, arms extended forward, into a smaller, more relaxed version.

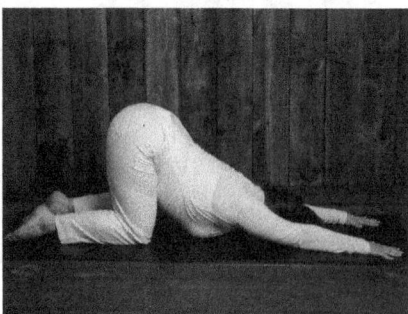

- If you prefer to deepen the heart opening qualities, you can opt to practise **Melting Heart Pose**. On your knees, arms reaching forward, like in puppy pose, but allowing the heart and rib cage to sink toward the ground, opening in the shoulders. You may want to prop your arms up on blocks or a bolster, or place a block to support your forehead.

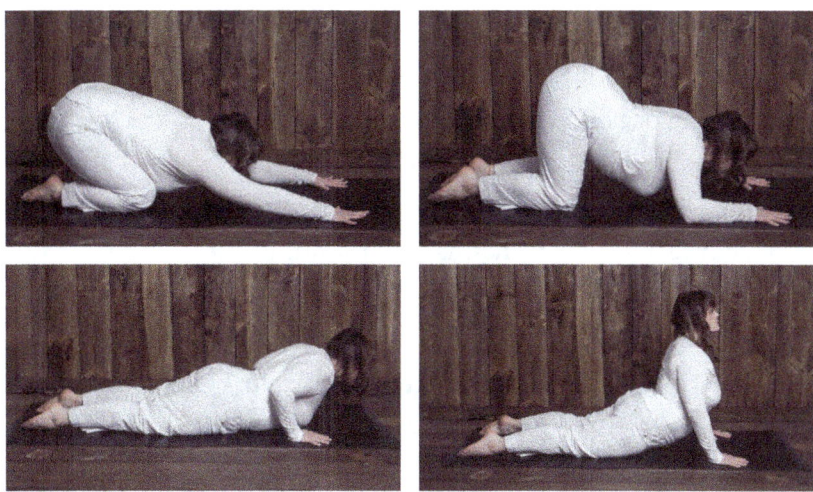

Child's Pose flow to Cobra: From Child's Pose, extend your arms forward, slightly wider than your shoulders, hands gripping the map lightly with spread fingers. Look between your hands, and keeping your heart near the ground, pull yourself forward as you extend your torso into a Baby or a Full Cobra Pose on your inhale. Exhale to return to Child's Pose. Repeat for a few breaths (approx. 4-8).

- Experiment with Bumble Bee (Brahmari) breath in child's pose. Inhale through the nose, exhale a humming sound, mouth closed, tongue on the roof of your mouth. This grounding breath helps stimulate the pineal gland;

often associated with the third eye chakra, developing intuition, and experiencing vivid or even prophetic dreams, it is physically responsible, namely, for the production of melatonin, essential in sleep regulation.

- For advanced yogi(ni)s and those with great body awareness, there's an option to take **Rabbit Pose (Sasangasana)**, after a brief resting period in child's pose (i.e., about four breaths). To take Rabbit Pose, place the forehead onto the mat, hook your feet with your hands, and rounding out your back, roll onto the top of your head, just beyond the hairline, keeping your neck long (no kinking!). Hold for a few breaths and on an exhale breath, return to child's pose. Rabbit Pose is a deep forward fold, rounds out the back, stretches of the west line of the body, and particularly behind the shoulder blades. In chakra yoga, Rabbit Pose is said to stimulate the crown, third eye, and heart chakras.

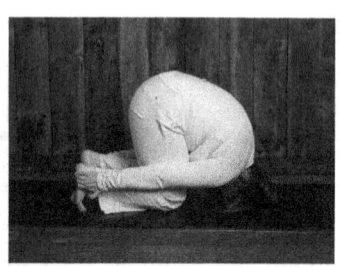

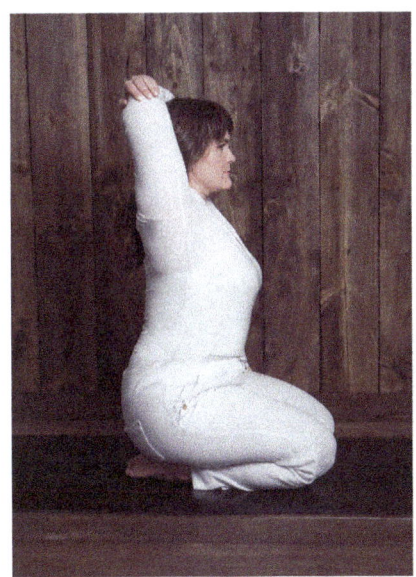 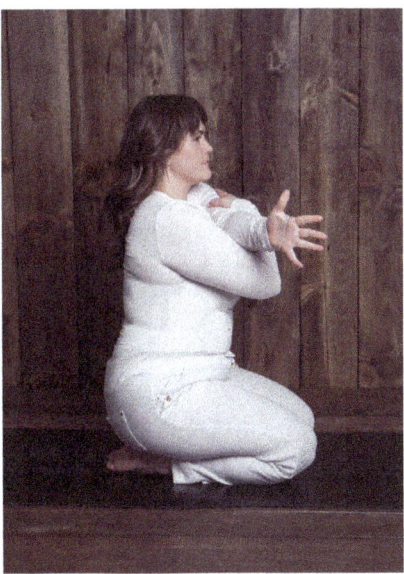

Rock pose + Toe Stretch: Sit on heels in rock pose, allowing a thigh stretch (quadriceps). You may want to sit on a block or bolster to reduce the intensity, and/or to ease the pressure on your ankles. You can also pad your ankles with a folded mat or blanket.

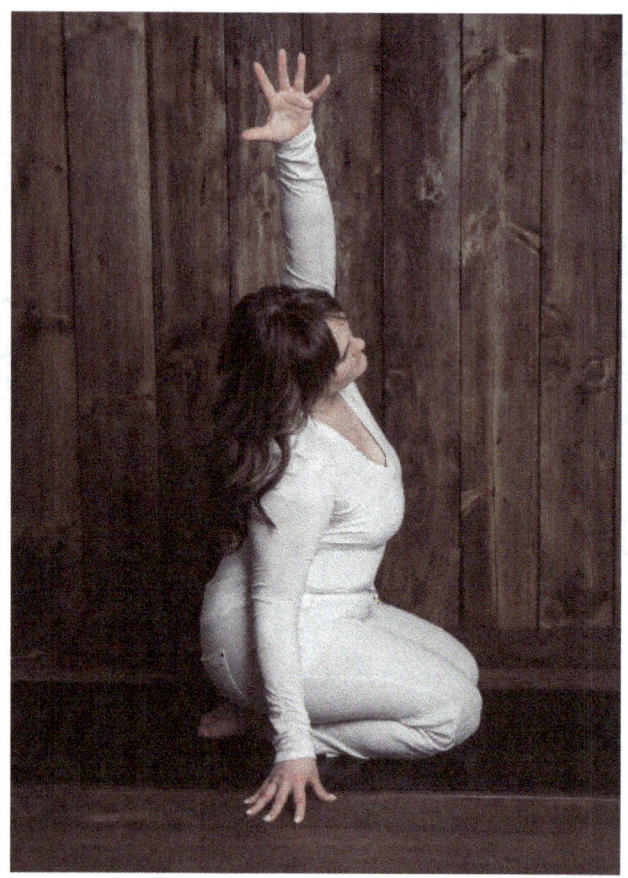

- Start from a neutral pelvis and extended spine, inhale in neutral, exhale into side stretches. You can move through these stretches and let your arms guide you overhead from side to side, while using one hand on the ground (or a block) on the bending side to control the intensity of the stretch.
- Tip: Your heart should face forward, not the ground.
- Check in with yourself. Offer a self-treatment of the chest, abdomen and back.

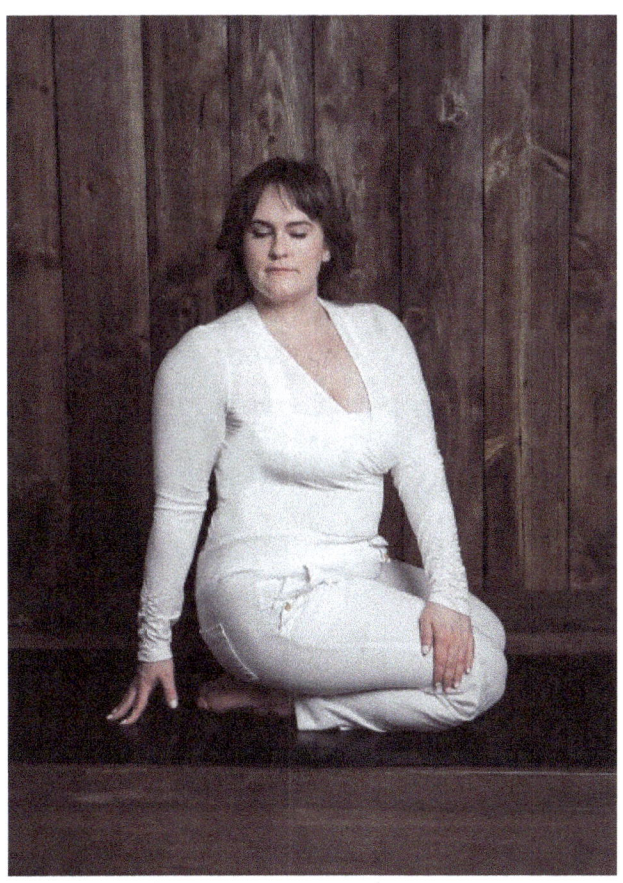

- Twist to either side, a hand on the ground behind you (or on your hip), and one hand on the outside of the thigh. Take a few breaths on each side.

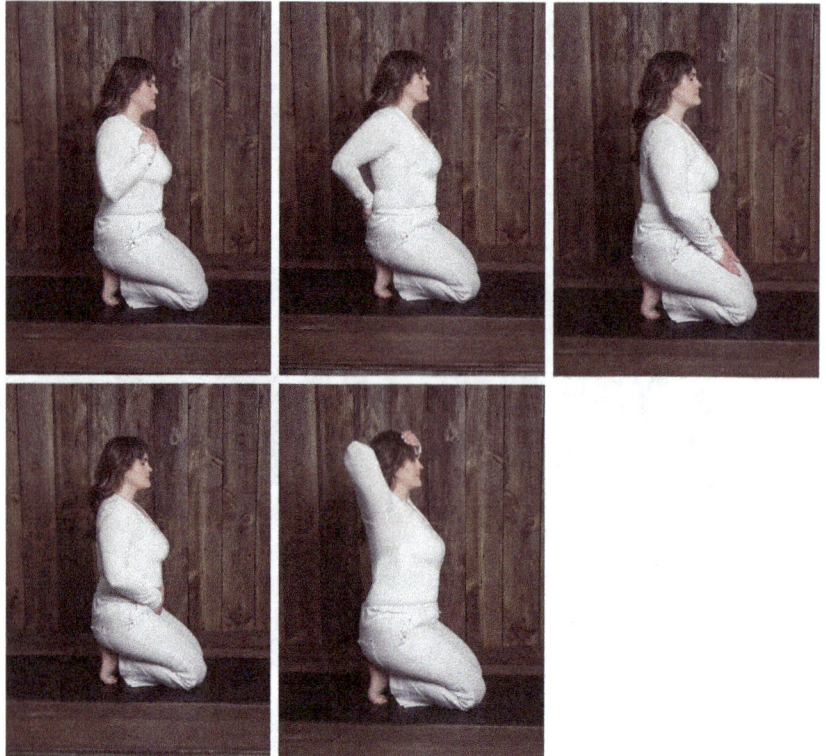

- Lift your hips off your heels, curl your toes under into toe stretch and lower the hips back toward your heels. You can sit on a block if it feels better for you.
- Place a hand on your heart and the other on your belly, giving yourself Reiki as you focus on your breath (approximately 4 – 8 breaths).
- Uncurl your toes, and find your way onto your belly.

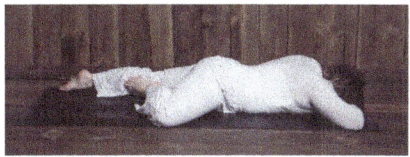 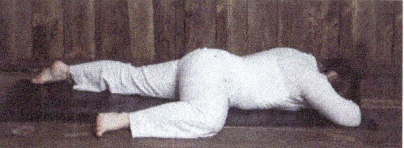

HALF (OR FULL) FROG POSE: Lying on your belly, draw your right knee up 90 degrees, shin parallel to your left leg, allowing your toes to point outward, with a flex foot. It looks like you might be trying to climb. Let your forehead rest on the back of your hands. You can opt for a "tree" modification if it feels better for you, by bringing the sole of your foot on the inside of your calf or thigh. Hold the hip opener for a few breaths, then do the left side.

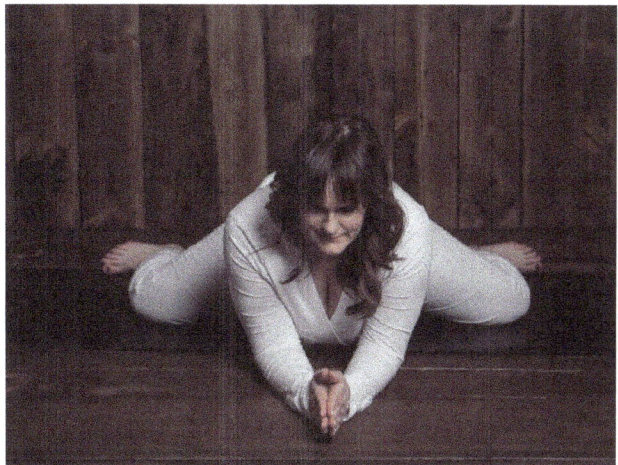

- Advanced option: you may choose to practise Frog pose, which requires proper alignment and possibly, torso support with a bolster so as to respect your current hip mobility.

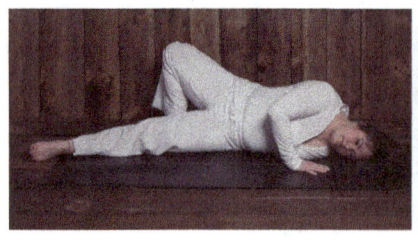 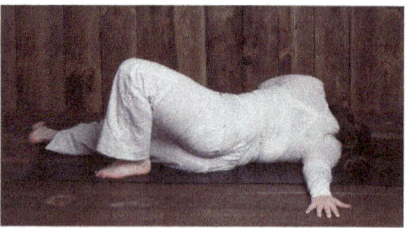

STAR STRETCH (OR BROKEN WING): On your abdomen, spread your arms in a T shape, palms down. Bring the left hand under the left shoulder and bend the left knee. Press into your left hand by keeping your right arm extended palm down, and gauge a comfortable stretch for the right shoulder. Place your left knee out to the side slightly to support your twist, or place your left foot behind your right leg for stability in the twist, whichever is most comfortable for your own back and torso. Let your head rest on a block, bolster, blanket, or the ground. Hold the pose for a few breaths. Release onto your belly for a breath or two, then do the other side. Turn onto your back when both sides are complete.

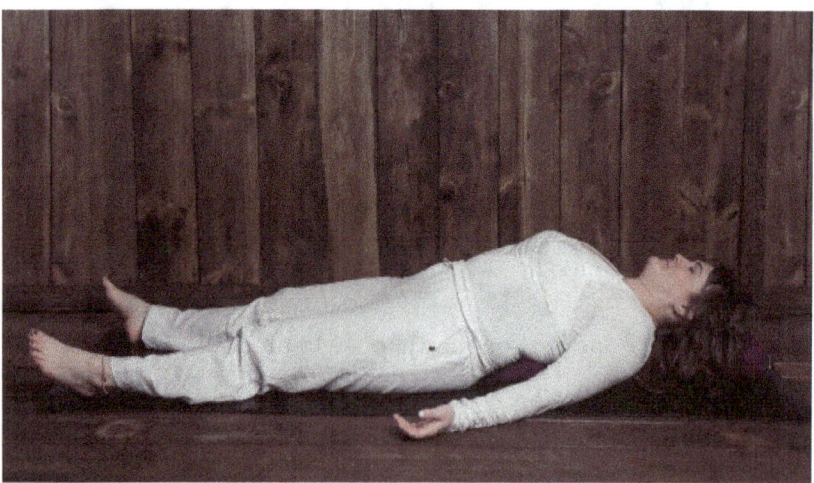

OPTIONAL HAND POSITIONS:

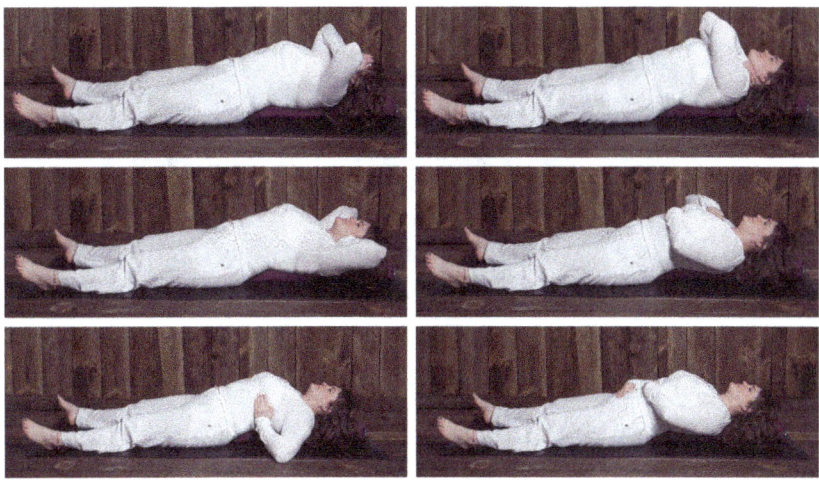

Supported Fish (Matsyasana): Using a bolster, thick rolled blanket, or two blocks, lie into Supported Fish Pose. If you are using a bolster or rolled blanket, place it lengthwise on your mat, at the bottom of your spine and lie onto it, allowing your arms to open on either side, palms up, and your heart and rib cage to "open." If the prop is too high for your body, causing lower back sensitivity or pain, adjust your props, and scoop your pelvis forward, away from the base of the bolster. If you are using blocks, place one width wise (especially if you have a short torso) under your heart (and allowing space for your shoulder blades to move above the block), propping your rib cage up. You may want to use a second block to support your head and allow your neck to rest into this pose.

- You can choose to simply rest here. You may choose to refocus on the Reiki pattern moving through your body, or offer yourself intuitive hand placements.

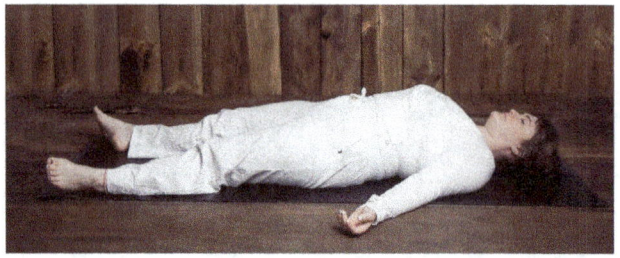

Savasana (integration/final meditation): lie comfortable on your back for integration of the practice and self-treatment.

USUI REIKI MANTRA OPTION: Hon Sha Ze Sho Nen

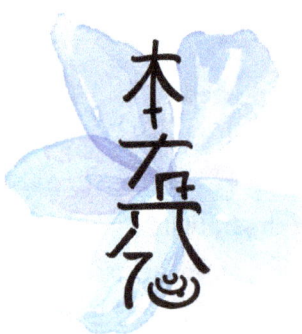

- You may wish to repeat a mantra before, during, or as you close the above Reiki yoga practice. Hon Sha Ze Sho Nen is a symbol Reiki practitioners use to facilitate energy healing through time and space, whether it is for personal reasons or to support others.
- It is particularly useful during distance Reiki sessions. Tapping into this symbol in mantra form activates the vibration of the symbol through toning (also called chanting).
- This is an excellent mantra to use when we are looking to break debilitating patterns, to dismantle negative family "traditions," to remove energetic blocks over time, or during a specific event.

YOGA MEDITATION OPTIONS:

- Kirtan Kriya – See Kundalini Healing Meditations Table

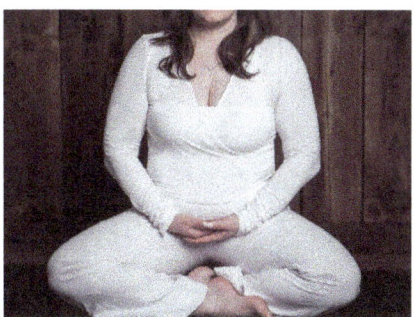

- Meditation for a neutral mind: In a seated position, opening with "Ong Namo Guru Dev Namo," place right hand into left, palms facing up, thumbs touching. Eyes closed, focus on the third eye point, repeat mentally the mantra "Wahe Guru" (from darkness to light) for 11 minutes (use a timer).

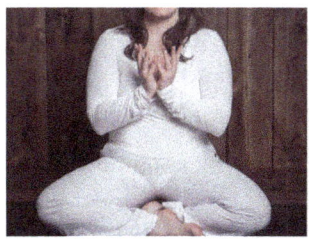 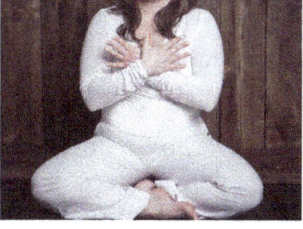

- **Padma mudra** (lotus), **Garuda mudra** (eagle)

Helpful meditations and mudras that support this type of healing and work on similar levels are the kirtan kriya, and the neutral mind, from the kundalini tradition. Lotus (padma) mudra and Eagle (garuda) mudra may also be helpful, as they respectively foster openness and freedom.

PART 3 HIGHLIGHTS

USE these sequences as they are to get you started, and feel free to build on them and make them your own.

Sequence 1 focused on **grounding** and worked physically on the legs and hips, as well as energetically on the Earth, base, sacral and solar plexus chakras.

Sequence 2 focused on **feeling** and worked physically on the back and torso, as well as energetically on the sacral, solar plexus, heart chakras, and on the Great (or 'etheric') Heart chakra.

Sequence 3 focused on **opening** and worked physically on the head, neck, shoulders, and arms, as well as energetically on the heart (and Great Heart), throat, third eye, crown and soul chakras.

These are gateway sequences to discovering the power of this practice that keeps on giving.

Part Four

The Journey

ENERGY HEALING MEDITATIONS

IN THE MONTHLY women's circle and group coaching I host from my BrightStarWoman.com website, we regularly meditate together. These meditations, all traditions combined, are some favourites.

MOTHER EARTH PINK HEART MEDITATION

When I need to feel unconditional maternal love and support, I practise this Mother Earth Pink Heart Meditation.

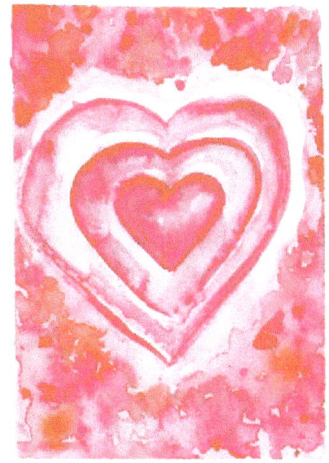

Lie down comfortably on the ground, either completely relaxed, or with one hand on your heart and one on the Earth. Observe your breath, letting yourself slow down and breathe deeply, balancing your in and out breaths. Connect with your own heartbeat through visualisation/feeling or using the hand you placed on your heart.

Visualize roots burrowing into the Earth to its pink lava core and ask respectfully to tap your energetic roots into the heart of the Mother. Breathe in Her rose, unconditional love, nurturing, and support through your roots back into your body. Then feel/see yourself filled and surrounded with Her light.

Feeling your steady heartbeat, wait to perceive/sense/feel/visualize Mother Earth's heartbeat synchronizing with yours. Feel you are One. Thank Her for her medicine, send Her love, and slowly untap your roots and bring them back into your body, knowing She is always there when you need Her.

BRIGHT STAR WOMAN - STAR HEART MEDITATION

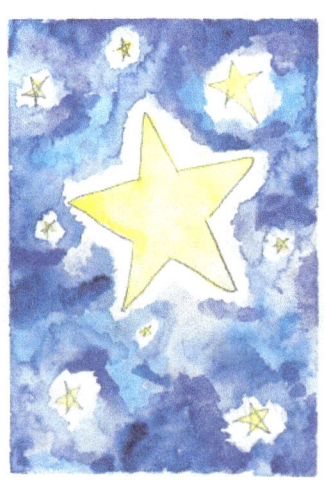

When I need empowerment and insight, and simply when I need to remind myself of the light being and powerful healer that I am, I practise my Bright Star Heart Meditation.

In a comfortable position, eyes closed, practise mindful breath, slowing down, breathing deeply (i.e., a count of four to inhale and four to exhale, or working up to more, from four to eight or more) allowing the exhale to be as long (or longer) than the inhale. This relaxes the nervous system.

When you feel present and relaxed, see your heart space filled with bright white shimmering light—it can even sparkle! With each inhale, the light brightens, and with each exhale, the light spreads outward to the rest of your physical and energy bodies. The light shines out from within like a star, until you are filled completely with light, until there's room only for wellness and peace. Practise this for several minutes, with or without a timer. When you feel ready, bring your awareness back to your body, introduce gentle movement, as you complete this meditation. You may choose to close with chanting, "Om shanti shanti shanti om."

KUNDALINI YOGA MEDITATIONS FOR HEALING

KIRTAN KRIYA – 11 MINUTES

Open: Ong Namo Guru Dev Namo

Time: 11 minutes (or 31 minutes for advanced meditators with an established practice)

Mantra: Sa Ta Na Ma

Posture: seated (cross-legged or on a chair, feet grounded)

Mudra: gyan, shuni, prithvi, buddhi

Breath: normal, as you chant the mantra (sung, spoken/whispered, silently)

Benefit: Balances all levels of consciousness and fosters healthy habits/behaviours, heals trauma (especially in women), supports addictions recovery.

Meditation: Visualizing an infinite beam of white light entering your crown and exiting your forehead, chant Sa Ta Na Ma, as you also produce the four mudras with each syllable. Sa is gyan mudra (index and thumb), Ta is shuni mudra (middle and thumb), Na is prithvi mudra (ring and thumb) and Ma is buddhi mudra (little and thumb). In the 11 minute version of this meditation, you will chant for the first 2 minutes, whisper for the following 2 minutes, silently repeat in your mind for 3 minutes, then resume whispering for 2 minutes and finishing by chanting for the last 2 minutes.

Tip: Use a timer with presets at the start, then at 2, 4, 7, 9, and 11 minutes to clearly signal when to chant, whisper, and silently repeat the mantra, and when to resume whispering and chanting.

Closing: Take a minute of silent meditation and mindful breath, then stretch arms overhead, fingers wide, and relax.

MEDITATION TO TRANSFER HEALING ENERGY

OPEN: Ong Namo Guru Dev Namo

Time: 1-5+ minutes

Mantra: silence

Posture: seated (cross-legged or on a chair, feet grounded)

Mudra: anjali (hands in prayer)

Breath: mindful, through the nose

Benefit: Supporting another's healing journey, cultivating positive vibrations.

Meditation: Press your hands together with strength as you visualize white light forming between your hands with each breath. Hold healing and loving thoughts in your mind and in your heart, as you intend to send these healing energies to a specific person, organization, or cause. Keep this up between 1 and 5 minutes.

When you are ready, use your breath to intentionally send the healing energy you've pooled to your recipient; send the light on your exhales. Some see a thunderbolt of energy being projected as they exhale. This is an energetic massage; you may choose to picture how the person is receiving it (perhaps gentler, or with more power). Some people prefer to keep their hands together, while others keep them together and point out, or open their palms out (fingers still together) as they visualize their recipient receiving the healing light. You can do this for 1 to 10 minutes.

Closing: Take a few deep breaths, release the mudra and posture.

MEDITATION FOR HEALING – 11 MINUTES

OPEN: Ong Namo Guru Dev Namo

Time: 11 minutes (or 31 minutes for advanced meditators with an established practice)

Mantra: Ra Ma Da Sa, Sa Say So Hung

Posture: seated (cross-legged or on a chair, feet grounded)

Mudra: elbows in, hands out, palms facing up.

Breath: normal as you chant

Benefit: An all-around powerful healing meditation

Meditation: Elbows in (hugging your ribs), place your palms up flat, fingers together like your holding platters. Visualize emerald green light flowing through and around you like a fountain of youth and healing. Chant Ra Ma Da Sa, Sa Say So Hung, and contract the navel to the spine on the "Sa" and the "Hung" syllables as the end of each phrase.

Closing: Inhale deeply and hold the breath, offer a healing thought. Visualize the person you wish to support as totally healthy and radiant; see your recipient as resilient and healed, as they are completely surrounded in a healing white light. Exhale, repeat once and exhale. Take a deep breath.

To explore kundalini healing meditations, read Meditation As Medicine by Dharma Singh Khalsa and Cameron Stauth, or consult 3ho.org

COMPLEMENTARY PRACTICES
WORKING WITH ENERGY

REIKI IS AN ENERGY-BASED PRACTICE; it is about tapping into life energy accessible to all, and honing the skill of channelling it for ourselves and to share with others (family, friends, near and at a distance, as well as clients and students). Learning to perceive, build, direct, and expend energy in a conscious and constructive way is crucial to improving the personal, and professional, practice of Reiki, and by extension, of Reiki yoga.

Yoga's *pranayama*, or breath work and exercises, is an effective and accessible method to tap into energy, our own and universal life energy, also called "prana." I believe pranayama to be an intrinsic, almost organic part of an established Reiki yoga practice.

If you like an interdisciplinary approach, which can be argued is the genesis of Reiki yoga, practising other energy-based modalities to develop your awareness of the flow of energy, and to fine-tune channelling and your own "brand" of energetic perception, will support your Reiki yoga practice. Modalities such as different types of Reiki, shamanic and healing practices and rites, and Eastern traditions such as tai chi and qi gong would also contribute to a depth of understanding and experience with energy.

That being said, I would caution against scattering your attention in too many directions out of curiosity (or even out of insecurity, feeling like an "imposter"). When dipping into several new practices, one runs the risk of "knowing" in surface while not mastering an in-depth understanding of a modality's teachings and losing the benefits of truly embodying the experiences you pursue.

HEALING THE FEMININE

As a Womb Keeper, I cannot recommend enough the gentle, yet potent, transformative power of the 13th Rite of the Munay-Ki, the Rite of the Womb.

The Rite of the Womb was channelled by Marcela Lobos and shared widely to help women heal their wombs, physically, emotionally and energetically. It is a practice, a feminine empowerment rite meant to clear the fear, pain, and trauma (of any kind, not exclusively of a sexual nature) that women may hold in their creative, life-giving matrix. In chakra speak, we would call it the space and energy of the sacral chakra.

"Munay" in Quechua means "love and will." The Japanese word "ki" means energy. Together, these words combine to mean "energy of love." The initiation rites of the Munay-Ki are rites of loving energy. There are 12 previous rites, usually acquired in apprenticeship or dedicated study; however, they are not prerequisites to this 13th rite. In fact, all Womb Keepers (recipients of the Rite, like me and thousands of other women) are encouraged to share the ceremony and healing energy with a sister who is ready to heal her divine feminine energy. She then can recreate harmony of the masculine and feminine, while embracing freedom, joy, compassion, and peace.

The Rite comes to us at a time of confusion where healing is greatly needed. We are all dual-energy beings; in all men, there is feminine energy, and in all women, there is male energy. In our modern Western culture, there is much imbalance in these energies. There are outbreaks of violence against women, increasing water pollution, and rising mental illness statistics, just to name a few of the concerning trends.

It is often a challenge to find one's place, to find peace inside ourselves. Especially when so much is vying for our attention. Many men struggle to find their identity as gender roles collapse. Many are taught unhealthy ways of relating to others and handling emotions (or just to suppress them altogether) and are faced with toxic masculinity ingrained in cultural practices. Actor and producer Justin Baldoni's web series *Man Enough* addresses this beautifully. Women are concerned about their safety on a daily basis in most of the world. Moreover, they often believe, consciously or unconsciously, that they must be more like men in order to succeed, to be worthy, to be "enough"...

Essentially, the 13th Rite of the Munay-Ki, the Rite of the Womb, is a rite meant to empower women and heal the feminine component of a woman's energy.

Menopausal women benefit from this rite as it assists them in the transition from their younger selves (the Maiden archetype) and their "fertile years" (the Mother archetype) into their wise years, transforming bodies and their associated strengths and emotions (the Crone or Wise Woman archetype). In the western world, we tend to only value women's youth and reproductive ability as feminine (but sadly, not her postpartum body), or even as the only desirable state, which is ludicrous!

Granted, culture can be a powerful influence on aging women's psyche, which is why fashion, beauty and plastic surgeries are multi-billion industries. If a woman can confidently and bravely face her aging self, she is rewarded with immense wisdom, freedom and healing power that she can enjoy and in turn, can inspire younger generations.

Women who've experienced reproductive organ cancers, other reproductive trauma, have had a hysterectomy or partial removal of the reproductive organs, may find this especially helpful to reconcile their concept of femininity, their emotions and their bodies with their experience and allow for them to move through complex energies into peace and acceptance. This is healing.

Though it is designed for women (born as women/identify as women) – the water bearers, men (born as men/identify as men) who wish to actively support the women in their lives, can do so by simply holding space during this ceremony. In this capacity, men are recognized as "fire keepers" and protectors.

My husband was present when I received my Rite from a trusted friend and his support was deeply appreciated. I have hosted this ceremony for groups of women as well as one on one. Seek and do what feels best to you.

That being said, some men (and fellow non-binary and transgendered people) will feel called to clear their sacral chakra, whether they have a physical womb or not, and adapt this Rite for personal needs and reasons. If you don't fall under the traditional definition of "woman," or do not have a womb, but feel called to receive this Rite, trust this nudge and explore this further, explore possible energy healing modalities that address the sacral chakra, and follow your guidance.

Visit my website, BrightStarWoman.com, and Marcela Lobos' site, TheRiteOfTheWomb.com, for more information on the Rite, how to receive and share it.

The Rite of the Womb supports reclaiming one's own healing power, with all that this entails, whatever this means to you: assertiveness, setting healthy boundaries, acceptance, receptivity, love, self-compassion, or simply being.

DEVELOPING INTUITION

Beyond a few guidelines, Reiki yoga is an intuitive process where trusting your body's messages, your gut instincts, and your own "brand" of intuition and/or extra-sensory perception is the modus operandi, the practice itself.

Meditation, of any tradition or school of thought, has been proven a cornerstone to mental health, self-awareness, personal growth, and spiritual connection.

The Emotional Freedom Technique (EFT) or "tapping" on pressure points as you speak difficult emotions with the intention of processing these emotions and breaking free of negative patterns, gives one a powerful tool to understand oneself and distinguish our reactions from our true selves.

Chakra Yoga is a practice where yoga poses, breathing, and meditations are meant to stimulate and balance the body's energy centres, supporting one's awareness and lived understanding of prana (life energy).

Journaling, which comes in many approaches, can foster self-awareness and emotional health. All of these awareness promoting methods are effective intuition catalysts.

CARING FOR OUR BODY

Though Reiki yoga is primarily therapeutic and gentle, caring for our bodies in complementary ways is important for holistic wellness. It's all too easy to fall into the trap of "not being a fitness person." Exercise, even low-impact activities like walking and stretching, contribute to cardiovascular, lymphatic, and tissue health. All of which are important for essential systems to function optimally, including our immune health and repairing damage in case of injury. Our bodies are our vessels and carry through our human experience; we can be spiritual people, but if we don't value the body we're given, we cannot experience holistic health, which is equally physical, mental, emotional, and spiritual.

I had a personal realization when I struggled with my hypothyroid condition that if I didn't invest more energy and care in supporting my body, it would not support me further on my spiritual journey. When that sunk in, I started embodying this understanding by making choices that were beneficial to my mental health, yes, but also to my physical health. I started sleeping earlier, eating fresher, going outdoors, walking more, and making meditation a daily habit.

MOVEMENT

It's important to note that there are "active" ways to care for yourself physically, like exercise (whatever approach lights you up, whether it's high-energy or gentle, as long as it gets you moving and makes you happy), as well as physically therapeutic modalities like Yoga Tune-Up™ and self-massage, as well as yin and restorative yoga. These latter examples contribute to tissue and joint health, and both claim an emotional component, as unexpressed emotions are logged in the body. Yin yoga, especially from a meridian focus (stemming from its genesis in Traditional Chinese Medicine [TCM]), approaches yoga postures from the organ health perspective and its subsequent emotional release. Self-massage is said to release emotions that may cause muscular and tissue tension and adhesions.

Another way to care for our bodies is through receiving care and healing modalities, like massage therapy, reflexology, acupuncture, physiotherapy, and chiropractic care, just to name a few.

NUTRITION

Naturally, nutrition is an essential aspect of body care as it fuels our functions physically and energetically. Foods contain physical nutrients but also energies. This may be an overly simplified example, but we can all agree that a fresh apple doesn't feel the same as a cooked one, and our bodies don't receive it in the same way either! Even without knowledge of nutrition, we know that a bowl of oatmeal does not digest similarly to a handful of nuts and a cup of fresh fruit.

Most personal trainers will tell you that "fitness is created in the kitchen." I know this to be true to a certain degree. I know incredibly healthy people who "never train," but eat sensibly and spend time outdoors, or simply practise gentle yoga. And there are certainly people who "hit the gym" and have a six-pack of abs who have toxic lifestyle habits.

I also know that the way you choose your foods, how you prepare them, the intention you choose when preparing meals, and how you feel about your food have an equal if not greater impact on both its physical effects as well as on mood (or its energetic effects).

Reiki practitioners will recognize here an opportunity to infuse foods with Reiki life energy to boost their nutritional value and their energetic benefits to the mental, emotional and spiritual bodies. Additionally, Reiki practitioners know that when Reiki flows through the body, it also helps it to absorb the best nutrients available, so Reiki and nutrition work collaboratively.

In essence, caring for your body will not only support you in your Reiki yoga practice, but in your creating holistic wellness, and in living intentionally, fostering greater meaning and satisfaction in your life and pursuits of all kinds.

AN ENVIRONMENT THAT SUPPORTS YOUR PRACTICE

THOUGH I AM no expert on home organization, minimalism, space clearing or feng shui, I have experienced first-hand how a space changes once it is energetically cleared with smudging and other shamanic practices. I also know that the recent (arguably, an ancient concept our ancestors knew all too well) "declutter and simplify" and minimalist movements have traction for a reason... because it shifts our whole lives by shifting our home-based energy! I have witnessed and experienced the transformation that happens when a home environment is decluttered, and it becomes a true reflection of who we are and how we wish to live.

Studies have shown that clutter exacerbates feelings of depression and anxiety. Some holistic wellness experts also link excess weight to hoarding tendencies (although that is an incomplete picture, it does invite reflection). A cluttered space is often akin to a cluttered mind.

However, everyone's definition of clutter and untidiness is personal, and each stage of our life requires different living circumstances. For instance, a young family will have greatly different needs from a single professional or a retired couple. Marie Kondo, whom I admire greatly, discusses the concept of "enoughness"—the point at which we feel we have the right number of things for any given category of possessions. For some, having five books may be enough while having a fully stocked kitchen with all the bells and whistles feels satisfying, whereas someone else may love their book collection, but choose a minimalist kitchen.

It's about values and priorities; your environment is a reflection of who you are and how you shape your life. If we approach our environment unconsciously, we often find ourselves overwhelmed by the mountain of stuff we accumulate, and perhaps bewildered by the things we choose to hold onto, and maybe even pulled in all directions emotionally, as past versions of ourselves call for our attention.

As an exercise in mindfulness, ask yourself how your space supports you being who you feel you are inside, and doing what makes you feel joyous and aligned. What do you love, what lights you up? Imagine walking through your front door at the end of the day, what do you want to feel, see, smell, hear, taste? How do you spend your time? Does your home reflect these preferences? If not, how can you make it happen?

Living a Reiki yoga lifestyle is about developing self-awareness and understanding energy, which becomes natural through practice. Reiki, yoga, and Reiki yoga practitioners value sacred spaces, and this often begins at home. Inevitably, with a dedicated practice, you will refine your perception of energy, whether it be personal, spatial, or otherwise. I like the idea of "editing" my home and my life, not for outsiders, but to allow me to live in alignment with my values and priorities. The energy of your home will probably shift, whether it happens concurrently with your practice, as a consequence of your own growth, or through a conscious effort. Moreover, high vibrational activities such as yoga, meditation, prayer, and space clearing (i.e., a traditional sage smudge or sound baths) elevate the energy of a space immediately and over time. In any case, remember that everything is a process.

Essentially, energy flows smoothly in a tidy, ordered space. The energy also feels lighter in a happy home, and we don't feel the need to hold onto objects that have outlived their purpose for us, that have become useless, unattractive, or broken. When we allow those things to remain in our homes, our safe havens, we are allowing the vibration they trigger in us to repeat itself over and over, every time we interact with that object. These small vibrational pulls add up and leave us feeling drained, leaving us with less energy to nurture the relationships and hobbies we love.

ENERGY CLEARING AND SACRED SPACE

From an energetic practitioner perspective, space clearing practices will support you both in the material process as well as on the emotional level and keep your energy up. I suggest adopting some type of energetic space clearing practice along with the physical journey of decluttering and optimizing ("smart sizing"). Space clearing is as important to do in your home and workspace, as it is to do for your person. Often, we call it "energy cleansing" when we speak of clearing our own energy. It's like showering (energy cleansing for ourselves) and cleaning your home (space clearing for our environments).

Burning sage in a sacred smoke has been demonstrated to be beneficial to one's health, but there are also other herbal medicines (in the traditional indigenous sense), such as cedar, sacred tobacco, sweetgrass, and palo santo in South America. When using plant medicines, please be informed of their appropriate use, and respectful of the ways the plants were collected.

As mentioned earlier, you can also clear space with sound, like clapping, shaking a rattle, tapping a drum, ringing bells or singing bowls. Singing with intention might also clear and harmonize beautifully.

Simpler ways to space clear, but these methods require mindfulness and ritual to be effective, are opening windows for airflow (and chi to move differently), sweeping (out the old energy that no longer serves), and generally cleaning your surroundings with non-toxic, Earth-friendly solutions and bringing nature indoors will shift the energy in your space.

These space clearing and energy cleansing practices are also useful rituals for creating sacred spaces for your Reiki Yoga and meditation practices, but also in order to create a sacred haven at home.

I recommend reading and applying the teachings from Marie Kondo's books, *The Life-Changing Magic of Tidying Up* and *Spark Joy*, or from *Sacred Space: Clearing and Enhancing the Energy of Your Home*, by Denise Linn. These books are gifts in a world where noise and clutter is the norm, and for people who deeply crave peace and joy.

THE ETHICS OF SHARING & TEACHING REIKI YOGA

IN WRITING THIS GUIDE, I am essentially stating that Reiki, and by extension, Reiki yoga, is our birthright. Knowledge truly is power, and the power and knowledge are within all of us. Everyone is intuitive, in some form or another, and that can absolutely be cultivated. Everyone deserves wellness and is capable of creating it from within through mindful practices and intentional choices.

I believe that we should all have a right to information and have access to the modalities and tools that enable us to heal, and live holistic lives of wellness, meaning and purpose.

I feel I should, however, offer a few notes about ethics around sharing and teaching Reiki yoga. You have a body, thus you can practise yoga. Reiki lives within you, thus Reiki is yours to channel. Much like yoga is an ancient practice accessible to all, and we are all free to foster our own personal, at-home practice, the Reiki modality of healing and wellness is available to all. However, there are dedicated students of each of these disciplines who choose to pursue their learning further with the intention of sharing these gifts with the world.

These professional teachers and healers invest their time, money and other resources into mastering their modalities and sharing them. This must be acknowledged and respected. Yoga teachers often study and practise countless hours, and often travel great distances to deepen their knowledge and improve their teaching. When a student attends their classes, workshops, trainings, and retreats, they are benefiting from and paying for the expertise this teacher has to offer, and the convenience of receiving it in the package the teacher has offered. There is great value there.

In past living conditions, the world's healers lived in communities where their needs were met by the community in which they lived, as their skills were recognized and therefore, they were supported materially. Today, most healers and teachers are self-employed or entrepreneurs, as societal structures have changed. They may practise a variety of healing modalities, to varying degrees of collective acceptance and understanding. The broad umbrella of healers and teachers can include energy workers, coaches, counsellors, alternative medicine practitioners, herbalists and nutritionists, authors and teachers, speakers, art therapists and facilitators, intuitives, and psychic readers. This is not an exhaustive list but gives an idea of just how many avenues healers may choose to share their gifts and teachings.

Unfortunately, healers (outside of allopathic medicine) are no longer recognized or prized community members whose roles are understood, valued, and therefore supported materially. It may even be argued that worldwide health care is in crisis and in desperate need of reform, particularly in North America.

Standards of care are not applied everywhere equally, care providers are overworked and desensitized, and the health care system is actually centralized into a sick care system, where an engorged system is constantly in reactive mode. Health care will hopefully decentralize and optimize as we empower ourselves to take responsibility for our own well-being, begin to value alternative medicines as preventative methods, and seek allopathic interventions when truly needed. That, however, is another matter altogether. Please understand that I am not promoting one approach over the other; I firmly believe that ancient and alternative traditions complement modern science and medicine. Each has their value and their place in holistic wellness. As far as I know, acupuncture can't save you from a serious, life-threatening car accident, but surgery generally isn't necessary to treat allergies, hormonal or digestive issues, for example.

Fortunately, the absence of the former community recognition and structure allows these healers and teachers the freedom to set their own boundaries around their work, and set new abundance rules that resonate with them. Many healers and teachers choose to pursue their calling part-time, for financial reasons or convenience, while others commit fully, with some level of material risk initially, and go on to build successful and prosperous careers thanks to perseverance and appropriate support.

The same applies to Reiki master teachers and practitioners and yoga professionals; their investment and dedication has led them to become experts. In the same way, a passionate yoga student can share some lessons with fellow enthusiasts, a Reiki yoga practitioner may share their discoveries. Or a yoga teacher who has no prior training in Reiki may wish to explore Reiki yoga.

Bear in mind, however, that though we are all teacher and student at different times, that there is value in dedication and expertise. Moreover, in the material world we live in, professional titles hold meaning. Titles imply that education and training was pursued, indicating commitment to a discipline, but also providing reassurance that the practitioner can offer services safely and ethically.

For this reason, and out of respect for both paying students/clients and for dedicated teachers and healers, I encourage you to pursue some training before adopting a professional title, whether it is of "yoga instructor," "Reiki practitioner," or "Reiki yoga teacher."

I would advise professional yoga teachers to pursue official Reiki training (attunement levels one through four, depending on the chosen Reiki lineage) before teaching Reiki yoga formally, because however simple the Reiki modality may be, it is steeped in culture and grounded in practice.

In line with the law of the energy we put out comes back to us, I believe in the importance of integrity. This sometimes means admitting our own limitations. I have often referred my students and clients to other teachers, professionals, and books when their questions were beyond my own realm of knowledge, experience or expertise.

I have stated when things I shared were still new to me, uncomfortable, or beyond my mastery. I have disclaimed when I did not have the title or training, and was sharing from a place of experience or exploration, rather than the position of an expert. It is okay to be a student, in fact it's quite exciting! Just have respect for the journey and for what lived experience has to offer.

PART 4 HIGHLIGHTS

IN THIS PART, we practised a few of Bright Star Woman's favourite meditations, including the **Mother Earth Pink Heart Meditation**, the **Bright Star Woman – Star Heart Meditation**.

We also practised a handful of classic **kundalini yoga healing meditations**, such as the kirtan kriya (Sa Ta Na Ma), the meditation for healing (Ra Ma Da Sa, Sa Se So Hung) and the meditation to transfer healing energy.

We explored **complimentary practices** to support your holistic wellness and enrich your Reiki yoga, and continue to **grow your intuition** and **master your energy**.

We discussed how a **supportive environment benefits our Reiki yoga practice as well as the importance of energy cleansing, space clearing and creating sacred space.**

Finally, we discussed the **ethics of sharing and teaching Reiki yoga,** and determined that intention, integrity, and safety are cornerstones when spreading the word on this practice.

LIVING YOUR REIKI YOGA

As you have learned in this manual, you now have powerful tools to support you on your holistic health and wellness journey. As with any method, particularly with alternative health practices, it is effective if used intentionally and consistently. Remember that practice makes progress, and done is better than perfect. It's far more beneficial to be practising and learning from doing things "imperfectly" or even forgetting steps, than it is to delay practice in order to do things impeccably. Start where you are, with what you have, and keep going.

Although I believe Reiki is accessible to anyone and you may only ever use Reiki yoga for yourself, I can't emphasize enough the value of training in Reiki (many styles and teachers are available, and trainings are also offered via my website BrightStarWoman.com) to develop your abilities and deepen your Reiki yoga practice. Please consider a Reiki level one attunement with a trusted Reiki master teacher of your choice. If you intend to share it with others, then I would highly recommend you pursue

Reiki levels two and three, depending on your chosen lineage. This more exhaustive formal training is especially useful if you plan to teach Reiki yoga professionally or to friends, or even treat friends and family with Reiki (in a non-yoga capacity). Cultivate personal and professional integrity and help raise the profile while maintaining the ethics of the Reiki profession by learning and training before sharing.

If you are truly called to share Reiki yoga, then please share it!

Gift this book to a loved one or tell a friend about it, and refer to the Bright Star Woman website for resources, a monthly circle, coaching, courses, and more.

The world needs more presence, light, love, and ultimately, healing. And if you can hold a flashlight, light a tiny candle, or be a lighthouse in the darkness, then do so. No matter how big or small you feel your impact might be. By taking care of yourself, you are already accomplishing something huge for yourself and making the world brighter; you are giving others permission to uncover their own light. Your living example is the greatest testament, whether you consciously choose to teach or not.

Continue to practise, practise, practise...! Reiki is experienced, first and foremost. Yoga is practical. Combining these age-old disciplines in Reiki yoga becomes an exercise in mindfulness and a journey of empowerment. Learn and explore, as you create a meaningful, healthful, harmonious life for yourself.

PRAISE FOR BRIGHT STAR WOMAN REIKI YOGA MANUAL

Unique and Fresh–A Reference for All Yogis and Healers!

"A unique and fresh approach!

Blending the healing practices of yoga and Reiki for total body, mind and spirit awareness and alignment is indeed, needed now more than ever on our planet.

Mercedes writes from the heart. It is through her own healing experiences and growth in self awareness that make this practical book a reference all yogis and healers should have on their shelf."

Mary-Anne Haupt
Usui, Karuna, Blue Star, Animal and Lightarian Reiki Master/Teacher
Owner of Heaven On Earth Healing Arts Centre
heavenonearthhealingarts.ca

A World of Empowerment–Deep Dive Into Your Self

"In her book, Reiki Yoga Manual, Mercedes Déziel-Hupé, also known as Bright Star Woman, invites practitioners and readers into a world of healing and empowerment using Reiki and yoga as complementary tools. Her vulnerability creates a safe container as she encourages and empowers people to tune into their own wisdom using these two powerful tools.

Mercedes writes in the same way she teaches - from the heart and in her authentic voice. She provides in-depth guidance that is accessible to the experienced and curious alike.

Her approach to healing is a bouquet of various practices and tools woven together, ancient and modern, offered together for contemporary life.

She draws upon her own healing journey to guide readers; she shares from a place of experience, passion, purpose and a genuine desire to support others on their journey of discovery.

Using word and image, Mercedes Bright Star Woman shines a light on Reiki yoga and complementary practices to help you find your way home, to Self from the inside out. Her approach is one that cultivates intentionality, which leads to meaningful choices and self-honouring habits beyond the practice mat.

If you are ready for a deep dive into your Self, this manual will guide you gently and hold space for you."

Tatiana Ishwari Nemchin
Life and Business Coach
Founder of Mouvement :: Yoga, Danse, Musique
studiomouvement.com, @tatiananemchin on Instagram

ABOUT THE AUTHOR

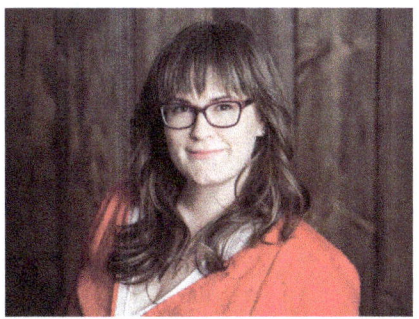

Mercedes Déziel-Hupé practised yoga for a few years before discovering its healing power in 2012 as a support to overcoming burnout and depression. Reiki helped Mercedes free herself from chronic anxiety and assist her mother as she was battling cancer. Reiki, yoga, and meditation together empowered her as she healed from medical conditions including hypothyroidism and a pre-diabetic condition, and heal from the grief of loss and later, from a traumatic birth experience.

Curious to reconnect with her indigenous heritage, she sought counsel and guidance from Elders and Wisdom Keepers of various nations. At 27, she received her spirit name, Bright Star Woman, which would confirm her path as a healer and teacher. The following year, the same Cree Elder who named her recognized her as Wolf Clan. As such, Bright Star Woman began a new journey as the bridge from ancient knowledge, wisdom and practices, to modern methods of healing and thriving in today's world.

Mercedes is a holistic life and wellness coach. In yoga, she specializes in a therapeutic approach, which translates into Reiki yoga, yin yoga, chakra yoga, gentle flow, and meditation. Through a variety of tools, from coaching to healing modalities, Mercedes holds space for her clients to tap into their personal power, helping them create harmony in body, heart, and mind.

Mercedes is a registered yoga and meditation teacher with the Yoga Alliance, Usui and Blue Star Reiki master teacher and keeper of indigenous rites, including the Rite of the Womb—the 13th Rite of the Munay-Ki. Accredited with the CTAA, Mercedes is a life coach, an EFT, NLP and hypnotherapy practitioner, a certified holistic nutritionist, and a reflexologist. She also holds a bachelor's degree in Communications and Philosophy from the University of Ottawa.

She lives in the National Capital Region with her husband and children, where she enjoys reading, dancing, watercolour painting, eating delicious whole foods, and paddling on flatwater.

REFERENCES FOR FURTHER EXPLORATION
WEBSITES REFERENCED

AUTHOR SITES:
Bright Star Woman Holistic Coaching
BrightStarWoman.com

Bright Star Woman YouTube Channel
https://www.youtube.com/@Brightstarwomanblog

ARTICLES:
12 Science-Based Benefits of Meditation, Healthline.com
https://www.healthline.com/nutrition/12-benefits-of-meditation

Rife Machines, CancerResearchUK.org
https://www.cancerresearchuk.org/about-cancer/cancer-in-general/treatment/complementary-alternative-therapies/individual-therapies/rife-machine-and-cancer

ORGANIZATIONS:

The Rite of The Womb
http://theriteofthewomb.com

The 3HO Organization, Kundalini Meditations
3HO.org

The Kirtan Kriya
https://www.3ho.org/kirtan-kriya

Sending Healing Thoughts Meditation
https://www.3ho.org/3ho-lifestyle/health-and-healing/sending-healing-thoughts-meditation

Ra Ma Da Sa Sa Say So Hung : The Ultimate Healing Tool
e-healing-tool

DOCUMENTARIES:

Heal, a documentary
http://www.healdocumentary.com/

Man Enough, Justin Baldoni's Web Series
Episode 1: https://www.youtube.com/watch?v=dVsbYas4tVo

Minimalism: A Documentary About the Important Things

BOOKS BY TOPIC

REIKI

Essential Reiki, by Diane Stein

Hands of Light, by Barbara Brennan

Karuna Reiki®, by Laurelle Shanti Gaia

Reiki Manual, by Penelope Quest

Shamanic Reiki, by Llyn Roberts and Robert Levy

YOGA

The Complete Guide to Yin Yoga: The Philosophy and Practice of Yin Yoga, by Bernie Clark and Sarah Powers

Yoga Anatomy, by Leslie Kaminoff and Amy Matthews

YinSights, by Bernie Clark

CHAKRAS

Chakra Yoga, by Anodea Judith

The Twelve Chakras, by Diana Cooper

Wheels of Life, by Anodea Judith

KUNDALINI MEDITATIONS

Meditation As Medicine, by Dharma Singh Khalsa, M.D. and Cameron Stauth

3ho.org

MUDRAS

Mudras: Yoga in Your Hands, by Gertrude Hirschi

MIND-BODY CONNECTION

The Anatomy of Spirit, by Caroline Myss

Eastern Body, Western Mind, by Anodea Judith

Light is the New Black, by Rebecca Campbell

Mantras in Motion, by Erin Stutland

Mind Over Medicine: Scientific Proof That You Can Heal Yourself, by Lissa Rankin, M.D.

NUTRITION

An Apple A Day, by Joe Schwarcz

Food As Medicine, by Dharma Singh Khalsa

Prescription for Nutritional Healing, by Phyllis A. Balch, CNC

WOMEN'S HEALING

Love Your Lady Landscape, by Lisa Lister

Rise Sister Rise, by Rebecca Campbell

The Inner Goddess Revolution, by Lyn Thurman

The Tapping Solution to Create Lasting Change, by Jessica Ortner

The Tapping Solution for Weight Loss and Body Confidence, by Jessica Ortner

The Way of the Happy Woman, by Sara Avant Stover

Warrior Goddess Training: Become the Woman You Were Meant to Be, by HeatherAsh Amara

Witch, by Lisa Lister

INDIGENOUS TEACHINGS

A Voice From the Wilderness, by Harry Snowboy

Kindling the Native Spirit, by Denise Linn

Medicine Woman, by Lynn Andrews

Shaman, Healer, Sage, by Alberto Villoldo

They Called Us "Savages" (On nous appelait les sauvages), by Dominique Rankin and Marie-Josée Tardif

ANGELS

A Little Light on Angels, by Diana Cooper

The Female Archangels, by Claire Stone

SPACES, ORGANIZATION, CLEARING, ENERGY

Sacred Space: Clearing and Enhancing the Energy of Your Home, by Denise Linn

Space Clearing A to Z, by Denise Linn

Spark Joy, by Marie Kondo

The Life-alternating Magic of Tidying Up, by Marie Kondo

MINIMALISM

Lightly, by Francine Jay

The Joy of Less, by Francine Jay

The Minimalist Home, by Joshua Becker

The More of Less, by Joshua Becker

The Year of Less, by Cait Flanders

You Can Buy Happiness: And It's Cheap, by Tammy Strobel

www.ingramcontent.com/pod-product-compliance
Lightning Source LLC
Chambersburg PA
CBHW071344080526
44587CB00017B/2957